# Access your online resources

*Working with Autistic Children and Young People* is accompanied by a number of printable online materials, designed to ensure this resource best supports your professional needs.

Go to https://resourcecentre.routledge.com/speechmark and click on the cover of this book.

Answer the question prompt using your copy of the book to gain access to the online content.

# Working with Autistic Children and Young People

This book focuses on appreciating the different language and communication style of autistic youngsters and discusses how therapists can respond to and support this to get the best out of their practice. Each chapter begins with a summary of key points and areas to focus on, includes "what to do" ideas and mini case studies to illustrate points, as well as signposting further reading. The book draws on relevant theory and offers practical insights to allow the therapist to develop confidence, knowledge and skills.

Topics covered include:

- Identifying effective support.
- Emotional regulation.
- Working with technology.
- Specific groups such as girls with autism.

Linking theory and practice in an engaging and easy-to-follow format, the book provides practical ideas that are immediately helpful for busy professionals to guide clinical decision-making and intervention. It is an invaluable addition to the toolkit of any speech and language therapist, as well as other professionals wanting an overview of how to work with autistic children and young people in our neurodiverse society.

**Sally Mordi** has worked as a Speech and Language Therapist since the 1990s. She has enjoyed varied roles with pre-school and school-aged children and young people in mainstream and specialist settings. She has been a clinical lead for autism in Enfield for more than ten years.

# The *Working With* Series

The *Working With* series provides speech and language therapists with a range of 'go-to' resources, full of well-sourced, up-to-date information regarding specific disorders. Underpinned by robust theoretical foundations and supported by intervention options and exercises, every book ensures that the reader has access to the latest thinking regarding diagnosis, management and treatment options.

Written in a fully accessible style, each book bridges theory and practice and offers ready-to-use and well-rehearsed practical material, including guidance on interventions, management advice, and therapeutic resources for the client, parent or carer. The series is an invaluable resource for practitioners, whether speech and language therapy students, or more experienced clinicians.

Books in the series include:

*Working with Communication and Swallowing Difficulties in Older Adults*
Rebecca Allwood
2022 / pb: 9780367524784

*Working with Solution Focused Brief Therapy in Healthcare Settings*
Kidge Burns and Sarah Northcott
2022 / pb: 9780367435097

*Working with Children Experiencing Speech and Language Disorders in a Bilingual Context*
Sean Pert
2022 / pb: 9780367646301

*Working with Global Aphasia*
Sharon Adjei-Nicol
2023 / pb: 9781032019437

*Working with Trans Voice*
Matthew Mills and Sean Pert
2023 / pb: 9781032012605

*Working with Autistic Children and Young People*
Sally Mordi
2023 / pb: 9780367723149

# Working with Autistic Children and Young People

## A Practical Guide for Speech and Language Therapists

**Sally Mordi**

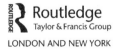

Routledge
Taylor & Francis Group

LONDON AND NEW YORK

Designed cover image: © Getty Images

First published 2024

by Routledge
4 Park Square, Milton Park, Abingdon, Oxon OX14 4RN

and by Routledge
605 Third Avenue, New York, NY 10158

*Routledge is an imprint of the Taylor & Francis Group, an informa business*

© 2024 Sally Mordi

The right of Sally Mordi to be identified as author of this work has been asserted in accordance with sections 77 and 78 of the Copyright, Designs and Patents Act 1988.

*British Library Cataloguing-in-Publication Data*
A catalogue record for this book is available from the British Library

*Library of Congress Cataloging-in-Publication Data*
Names: Mordi, Sally, 1974- author.
Title: Working with autistic children and young people: a practical guide
for speech and language therapists/Sally Mordi.
Description: Abingdon, Oxon; New York, NY: Routledge, 2023. |
Series: Working with | Identifiers: LCCN 2022058337 (print) | LCCN 2022058338 (ebook) |
ISBN 9780367723156 (hardback) | ISBN 9780367723149 (paperback) |
ISBN 9781003154334 (ebook)
Subjects: LCSH: Autistic children-Language. | Autistic children-Means of
communication. | Speech therapy. | Speech disorders in children.
Classification: LCC RJ506.A9 M667 2023 (print) | LCC RJ506.A9 (ebook) |
DDC 618.92/85882-dc23/eng/20230417
LC record available at https://lccn.loc.gov/2022058337
LC ebook record available at https://lccn.loc.gov/2022058338

ISBN: 978-0-367-72315-6 (hbk)
ISBN: 978-0-367-72314-9 (pbk)
ISBN: 978-1-003-15433-4 (ebk)

DOI: 10.4324/9781003154334

Typeset in Interstate
by Deanta Global Publishing Services, Chennai, India

Access the Support Material: https://resourcecentre.routledge.com/speechmark

# Contents

# Figures

# Tables

# Tables

# Background

SECTION II
Background

# INTRODUCTION

DOI: 10.4324/9781003154334-2

# Introduction

This book is designed to be a practical guide for therapists who want an overview of how to work with autistic children and young people in our neurodiverse society. The emphasis is on appreciating the different language and communication styles of autistic children and young people and supporting the people in the youngsters' community to understand, accept and appreciate their perspective. Where autistic children and young people have additional language and communication needs, the focus is on identifying effective support.

As you go through the book, you will find practical "what to do" ideas and resource recommendations alongside (anonymised) mini-case examples to illustrate points. It can be used alongside the RCSLT Autism Guidance due to be published in summer 2023 (www.rcslt.org) which reviews and updates RCSLT resources and information about autism and the role of speech and language therapy.

---

### TERMINOLOGY

Terminology remains controversial: "person with autism" versus "autistic person." The person first, "person with autism," highlights the need to think about the person rather than the autism. This originated from a desire to be more respectful of the person and avoid language that was felt at that time to be derogatory. However, many autistic people prefer "autistic," considering their autism as a fundamental part of themselves and recognising the difference, not deficit. Not everybody agrees, and not all individuals can express their opinion, although the arguments are powerful. Where possible, ask the child/young person what they prefer.

Autism is a complex condition, and this is reflected in the terminology. Most recently, the *Diagnostic and Statistical Manual of Mental Disorders, Fifth Edition* (DSM-5; American Psychiatric Association, 2013) has specified the term **autism spectrum disorder** (ASD); and the *International Classification of Diseases, 11th Revision* (ICD-11; World Health Organization, 2018) uses the same terminology. ASD reflects the deficit-based medical diagnosis. Here, "autism" is used for all autism spectrum disorders. Many autistic adults challenge the idea that autism is a disorder.

Neurodivergent is an inclusive term that reflects the view that brain differences underlie autism and other neurodevelopmental diagnoses. This evolves from the social model of disability: disability results from societal barriers rather than individual differences. Neurodiversity includes everyone; neurotypical describes people with a brain that develops and functions in a way that is considered typical. Neurodivergent describes people with a brain that works differently from that considered typical.

"Autistic people have a unique set of characteristics, which can manifest as difference, disability, or gifts/skills, from person to person and within the same person" (Autistic Self Advocacy Network, 2015).

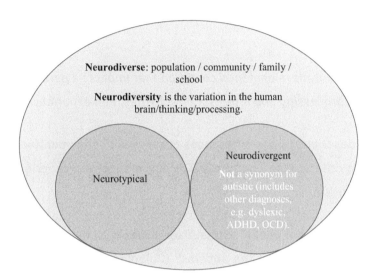

**FIGURE 1.1** Neurodiversity terminology.

The speech and language therapist (SLT) works as part of a team with the child who has (or might have) autism. The makeup of this team will vary but will include at least the family and education/early years setting. The skill mix of the team can be highly varied depending on the stage and setting. The team must work together to ensure that the support is integrated.

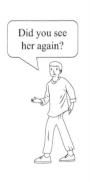

As a relatively newly qualified SLT, I met John. He was a bright and thoughtful eight-year-old boy. John attended the language unit attached to the mainstream school where I worked. He responded well to learning in a small group, with lots of focus on social communication. One Monday morning, he listened attentively as all the staff and pupils reported their news. Mine had been of a friend standing on the toilet painting the ceiling. The toilet seat broke, and she fell into the loo. John's facial expression remained impassive as usual while the other children laughed. He later quietly approached me and asked, "did you see her again?" He was extremely relieved that she had only wet her foot.

John was one of the first children I met with significant social communication difficulties (at the time, he did not have a diagnosis of autism). His learning style was confusing: he was articulate but often did not understand. Over the last 25 years, I have worked with many children and young people, their families, teachers, support staff, doctors, therapists and psychologists. Autism has become more familiar and better understood, but challenges remain as the neurotypical world is confusing.

## What is autism?

*Autism is a lifelong, neurodevelopmental condition that impacts a person's social communication, information processing and interests or activities, and experience of the world.*

Autism is usually described by the **differences** observed in behaviour and often with reference to diagnostic criteria (see Chapter 2). Our knowledge and experience influence our understanding of autism.

The considerable diversity of people with autism makes it a challenge to be more specific in describing autism succinctly. "The autisms" (Coleman & Gillberg, 2012) is sometimes used to reflect the variable nature of autism, which is likely to be more clearly defined in the future with different subtypes.

## An extremely brief history

Kanner and Asperger first wrote about autism in the 1940s. Parent and psychiatrist Lorna Wing wrote the acclaimed text, *The Autistic Spectrum* (Wing, 1996), having developed the idea of autism as a *spectrum* which has included more people. Currently, the prevalence of autism is around 1.8% of people in the United Kingdom (Roman-Urrestarazu et al., 2021). About 50% of people with autism have learning difficulties (National Autistic Society, 2018). More recently, the "autism constellation" has been used to highlight the change in our understanding of the multidimensional profile seen in people and in an individual at different times (Hearst, 2022).

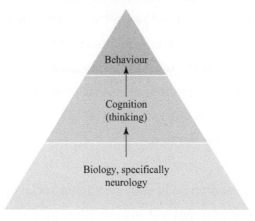

**FIGURE 1.2** Observable differences in behaviour resulting from differences in biology and cognition.

See *Neurotribes* (Silberman, 2015) for a comprehensive historical perspective.

Psychologists Fletcher-Watson and Happé (2019) helpfully describe autism in terms of differences in behaviour observed, and differences in both cognition (thinking) and biology.

Behaviour: we can <u>observe</u> differences in the following:

- Response to **sensory** experience,
- **communication** and **interaction.**
- Intensity of **interests** or **activity** and **information processing.**

This can look very different from one autistic individual to the next and at different life stages. No behaviours are unique to autism; a neurotypical person (i.e. a person who does not have a neurodevelopmental disorder) may have behaviour that appears "autistic," but it is the pattern and intensity of the behaviours that are significant.

> "If you've met one person with autism, you've met one person with autism," attributed to Stephen Shore, autistic professor of special education at Adelphi University, New York.

A diagnostic assessment considering autism focuses on observable behaviour. Fletcher-Watson and Happé's description helps focus attention on the reasons for the behaviour. This is useful in identifying what support could help.

Cognition (differences in thinking): an autistic person will experience the world differently. For example, there are differences in information processing and understanding, and sensory processing and integration. There are theories about the cause. While these can help understand some of the differences observed, no one theory explains the wide range of differences in people with autism.

Biology: genetic variations are often associated with autism. Neuroimaging (e.g. magnetic resonance imaging [MRI] scans) shows specific differences in neurology. For example, there is often an observable difference in an infant's brain: despite typical brain size at birth, scans in the second year of life show overgrowth that precedes an autism diagnosis (Girault & Piven, 2020). At present, no differences seem to have been identified in neurological anatomy or function that are consistent for all people with autism.

> Prizant described autism as a "disability of trust" (Prizant, 2019) with an impact on:
>
> - Trusting the person's own **body**, often as a result of sensory differences.
> - Trusting the **world**, which is unreliable (e.g. batteries run out, roads get closed).
> - Trusting **people** who are unpredictable and inconsistent.
>
> These will have an impact on an individual's (emotional) regulation.

## Observable differences

## Differences in social communication/interaction

The <u>autistic pragmatic language hypothesis</u> (Cullen, 2021) proposes that autistic people possess a "unique functional pragmatic system," which is different rather than deficient. It is characterised by:

- Literal processing: prioritising semantic meaning, irrespective of social context.
- Word, rather than sentence level, meaning interpretation, so Cullen proposes that the processing load is higher than for neurotypical people.

This hypothesis may explain some of the communication differences.

*Spoken language, which may include*

- No, or extremely limited, use of spoken language.
- Advanced language skills at a young age.
- Vocabulary acquisition may be different:
  - May be highly advanced, especially relating to the child/young person's interests (e.g. use of specialised or technical language – "it's not a bee, it's a yellow-legged Asian hornet!"). Despite this skill, the youngster may have difficulties recalling familiar people's names.
  - May have a specific difficulty with the language of emotions (alexithymia).
  - Where the child's language skills are not so advanced, their vocabulary is typically stronger on objects (nouns) and relatively weaker with people (names) and actions (verbs).
- Professorial style of information sharing, demonstrating knowledge, persistence and (may be one-sided) engagement, often around own interests (associated with sophisticated vocabulary): sometimes referred to as "info-dumping" or "monologing"; these may be preferred conversational styles.
- Pronoun reversal: confusion using me/I and you, and/or child referring to their self (and sometimes parents) by name.
- Echolalia: immediate or delayed. Language can give clues about the young person's thinking: for example, using a learned phrase heard in a familiar situation to express self at a later date, may be incongruous, i.e., a child asking "have you washed your hands?" to an adult offering them fruit may be misinterpreted as rude, but could be a comment that hands are washed, a prompt that they need to wash their own hands or an expression

of anxiety. Echolalia can be used lifelong communicatively (see Chapter 5). When used by an autistic youngster, echoing generally imitates the prosody of the speaker, rather than changing this to reflect the response (e.g. rising intonation for a question "do you want juice?" "want juice?" as an affirmative, but sounds like a question).

- Unusual prosody, e.g. inflexible or particularly expressive prosody, may have an accent that does not reflect where they live.
- Other speech and/or language delay/disorder (language disorder can occur with autism).
- Processing speed (of language) may appear slower (particularly as social demands increase). A child/young person may be processing much <u>more</u> information than peers.
- Working memory (keeping in mind and using multiple pieces of information) may be affected.
- May use text to communicate as an alternative or a supplement to speech. May prefer communication that allows for time to think and respond (e.g. text, email, video messaging) rather than instant/live communication (preference for asynchronous communication).
- May be hyperlexic: with a sophisticated, self-taught ability to read (which may or may not be accompanied by an understanding of the text).

---

Ash had no speech, but moulded letters in playdough at his nursery to check the day's routine.

Zayn opted to write when responding to questions with an emotional aspect, rather than speaking.

---

*Responding to others*

- May not respond to own name (parents may wonder if their child has a hearing impairment).
- May show a lack of conventional (i.e. neurotypical) response to smile/facial expression/ feelings.
- May not respond to body language/gestures in neurotypical way.
- May respond in a different way than the expected way to bid for interaction from others.
- May have an excellent ability to attend to own interests. The child may not initiate or respond to attempts to share interests (joint attention) in conventional ways. For example, limited, absent or unusual looking between an item and person; may not follow another person's eye gaze, or follow and use a conventional point gesture, e.g. looking at the other person's hand, not the object in a distance point. May share interests by being alongside a peer.

- May (or may not) recognise someone unusually, for example, based on a single feature (e.g. glasses, hairstyle or an item of clothing).

> John asked of a familiar staff member, "who's that lady in the skirt?" He had consistently recognised the person when they wore trousers.

- Literal understanding, thus can find neurotypical ambiguous or non-literal language challenging. This can be subtle: the child/young person may answer the question, missing the implied request (e.g. *do you know where the scissors are?* "yes"); they may not understand different meanings signalled by intonation, which is often associated with a lack of awareness of the social situation (e.g. what are **you** looking at? "your eyebrows") or may misinterpret the language (PTO on a piece of paper, with lots of wriggling... "I can't I'm not lying down"). This can result in unusual responses and sometimes behaviour that is unexpected or challenging to others, but **when considered from a literal point of view, their answer is reasonable.**
- May have a sincere and non-judgemental response to others.

*Interacting with others*

- Interaction may appear to be to request/meet needs rather than social purposes. Use fewer points or "show" gestures.
- Conversations are likely to be focused on interests rather than neurotypical conversational starters (e.g. British weather, football, TV, weekend). Individuals may take on the speaker role, sharing their expert knowledge, so the conversation lacks flow from a neurotypical perspective. Conversation between autistic participants often has much longer turns.
- Social language may feel relatively learned/inflexible.
- Difficulty talking about emotions can have an impact on relationships.
- May have different awareness of personal space.
- May have different interests and/or approaches to others (e.g. initiation may appear over-affectionate or assertive).
- Play may be happy, relaxed and purposeful with their preferred activity. May find pleasure in repeating the same play sequence.
- May play alone or alongside peers. Any social play may appear passive or rather assertive.
- Friendships may be determined by recognising a peer's skills in an area of particular interest (e.g. friendship based on identifying a peer as a great train track engineer). Girls are more likely to initiate friendships but may have more difficulty maintaining the relationship. Friendship may be with a younger or socially less sophisticated peer.

- May not appear to share enjoyment with others (e.g. reduced, unusual or absent eye contact, smile, pointing).
- May not compensate for lack of language using conventional means with gestures and/ or facial expressions.
- Coordination of non-verbal cues (e.g. facial expression, eye contact, body language) may be reduced or unexpected.
- May appear to use a person as a tool (e.g. leading an adult to a locked door by their key fob to access a preferred item).
- Literal interpretation of situations. Other (neurotypical) people may interpret this as unusual or (inappropriately) assertive.
- May develop very close relationships extremely quickly.
- Likely to be very loyal within relationships.

## Differences in information processing, interests and activities

- Play may be focused on a particular preference.
- May demonstrate imaginative play relating to interests.
- Stimming: repetitive movements (e.g. hand flapping, rocking, spinning, finger flicking), which often help with regulation or may be enjoyable.
- May have an intense interest: extremely skilled and/or knowledgeable, could be unusual in content. Interests, particularly of girls, may appear typical, but when explored, an unusual quality of and/or intensity in the interest is apparent.
- May have considerable creative talents.
- May have a strong need to follow their own agenda and difficulty with change and transitions (e.g. resistant to taking a different route to school, coping with unfamiliar situations).
- Focus on detail: very accurate, a good memory for facts and figures.
- A different perspective can result in remarkable insights and problem-solving.
- Organisation abilities may differ: highly organised (possibly also relatively inflexible) or appear disorganised.
- May have difficulty planning and/or imagining the future or may be highly competent but inflexible.
- May need help with generalising and thinking flexibly.

## Sensory differences

- May be over or under-responsive to sensory information (e.g. extremely sensitive hearing).
- May find it extremely difficult to ignore sensory information that appears insignificant to neurotypical people (e.g. labels on clothes, radiators gurgling, lighting).

- May have specific food preferences and/or a very limited diet (often able to detect minimal differences, e.g. a change in a recipe from a "safe" food or an attempt to disguise more variety).

- May appear to have an unexpected, extreme or reduced response to bodily sensations. This has an impact on the individual's recognition and expression of their feelings (e.g. need to use a toilet, thirst) and their emotions (e.g. difficulty sensing and interpreting fast heart rate and "butterflies" sensation as anxiety).

**Anxiety is a frequent consequence of navigating a neurotypical world that does not accommodate autism.**

---

With support to identify and talk about internal feelings, Hannah could identify, talk about and respond to how her body feels when she is starting to become dysregulated. This allowed her to begin to use strategies to regulate her emotions effectively.

---

Autumn did not experience pain in a typical way. She walked on her broken leg without complaint until her mother noticed her unusual gait and swelling and took her to the doctor.

---

**Cognitive:** some theories attempt to explain autism, but to date, no single theory does so comprehensively. However, they can help us understand behaviour, which allows us to know what support may be helpful.

*Theory of mind* describes our ability (or not) to think about our own and other people's mental states (e.g. their knowledge, beliefs, preferences and intentions) and use this information to understand and predict behaviour. This has an impact on social communication.

Many people with autism have difficulties with *executive functions*. These mental skills include working memory, flexible thinking and self-control. Autistic children and young people often have executive function difficulties, but they are not specific to autism; they are particularly prevalent in attention deficit hyperactivity disorder (ADHD). Competence in executive function (e.g. good planning, working memory and flexibility) may help a young person manage at home, school and in the community, but this may also make diagnosis and the identification of support more challenging as these skills may mask/camouflage difficulties experienced by the young person.

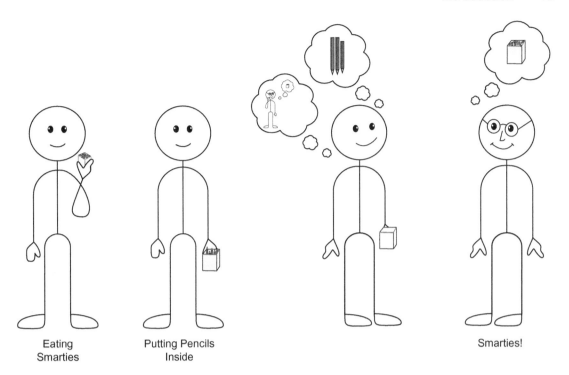

Eating
Smarties

Putting Pencils
Inside

Smarties!

**FIGURE 1.3** Theory of mind. Louis has eaten the smarties, filled the smartie tube with pencils and offered it to his friend. His friend thinks the tube is full of smarties. Louis knows it is full of pencils but knows that his friend thinks it is full of smarties. Where theory of mind is lacking, Louis would think that his friend thinks the tube is full of pencils (because he knows it is), a false belief.

Some theories focus on *early development*. They describe differences in attention and/or motor skill that have been observed in infants (of less than one year) who go on to be diagnosed with autism. These are usually research participants who are younger siblings of a child with autism.

It has been proposed that a very early difference in attention to social situations (where social information may not be so innately rewarding to infants who go on to have a diagnosis of autism) results in the child having less exposure to social/language learning situations. This may be a factor in language, interaction and social communication differences. Despite this, at the time of writing, there is no firm evidence of social, behavioural differences in infants' social responses.

Non-social early markers appear to be more robust. For example, differences in attention switching and motor development, including eye movements (e.g. sustaining looking for shorter periods in infancy), are associated with an autism diagnosis later.

There is evidence that autistic people often have differences in attention focus and/or sensory perception. This has led to information-processing theories of autism, including:

- *Monotropism*: a narrow focus of attention or attention tunnel (e.g. as if looking through a telescope), attending to a single or a few items (may be visual attention and/or other senses, e.g. hyperacusis: noise sensitivity). This can lead to highly developed knowledge, skills and analysis in the area of focus.

- *Central coherence*: weak central coherence describes the ability to focus on detail at the expense of the whole context. There is an argument that measures of the entire context could be biased towards considering social context, so any difficulty could be with the social aspect of the task rather than the whole context.

The *double empathy problem* (Milton, 2012) provides an alternative account of autism. It is compelling: it reframes autism as a problem for both autistic and non-autistic participants in an interaction. The miscommunication of the neurotypical person (e.g. using ambiguous language and/or assuming prior knowledge) causes the difficulties experienced. This may be at least as problematic as any perceived deficits of the autistic person in any challenges encountered by either person. Milton highlights the stigma and oppression from seeing autism as a pathology needing intervention, particularly where autistic people have historically been described as lacking empathy. He summarises: "One could say that many autistic people have indeed gained a greater level of insight into NT [neurotypical] society... than vice versa, perhaps due to the need to survive and potentially thrive in a NT culture" (p. 886). Neurodivergent people are "different, not less" (Fletcher-Watson & Happé, 2019).

## Useful resources

YouTube: An introduction to monotropism (Rose, 2022a)

YouTube: An introduction to the double empathy problem (Rose, 2022b)

## Biology: neurology/genetics

Work on genetics has shown that more than 100 genes are often associated with autism. Research is ongoing, and there are various theories about how genetic variants cause autism. Mostly there is no clear cause–effect relationship between specific genetic anomalies and autism. A possible explanation is that the individual has a *combination* of genetic variations, which may be common and/or rare (Wiśniowiecka-Kowalnik & Nowako, 2019). This could explain why there is an association between some relatively rare genetic mutations (e.g. Fragile X) and autism. However, not everyone with Fragile X has autism, so additional genetic variation, epigenetic or environmental factors may be involved.

The genetic influence on autism can be **inherited**: autism occurs more often in some families. For example, if one child in a family has autism, the likelihood of the next child having autism increases to about 10%. If two or more children have autism, the possibility of a subsequent child being autistic is approximately 33% (Ozonoff et al., 2011). In some families, there is evidence of some features of autism in relatives who do not fulfil the diagnostic criteria (broad autism phenotype or subclinical autism).

Alternatively, a **new mutation** may result in genetic changes associated with autism. There are several known syndromes where the genetic mutation is associated with an increased likelihood of autism (e.g. tuberose sclerosis, Fragile X, neurofibromatosis type1 [NF1]).

---

Aaron's skin markings were noticed by his GP incidentally when he attended for another issue as a toddler. He was referred to a paediatrician and diagnosed with neurofibromatosis type1. His parents were provided with information about a local support group for NF1. He started at his local school but struggled to settle, finding the social demands of a reception classroom extremely challenging. His understanding of spoken language was generally within the expected range, but he had some speech immaturities. Aaron constantly misinterpreted social situations, and despite being superficially chatty, he could not express his side of the problems. His teachers and SENCO tried to support him, but he was disruptive, and the school quickly initiated statutory assessment of his special educational needs. As part of this, he was seen by several professionals and referred to the diagnostic team. He was finally diagnosed with autism.

---

## Neurodiversity

In *The Real Experts: Readings for Parents of Autistic Children*, autism is described as "a genetically-based human neurological variant" (Walker, 2015). Supporters of the neurodiversity model propose that autism is "simply part of the natural spectrum of human biodiversity, like variation in ethnicity or sexual orientation… Ultimately, to describe autism as a disorder represents a value judgement rather than a scientific fact" (p. 12). This is an important perspective, although the view is not universal, particularly among families of children and young people with more than one diagnosis (e.g. learning disability and autism).

## Causes of autism

Causes of autism are usually described as being *genetic* or *environmental*. As research progresses, it is also clear that environmental and genetic factors can influence each other:

*epigenetics.* This is being actively researched to further investigate the interactions and their impact on individuals. For many people, autism is likely to result from genetic susceptibility and environmental triggers.

One model summarises how genetics, epigenetics and environmental factors may interact. Environmental factors influence gene expression (epigenetics) before conception and in the prenatal environment. These interact with the infant's genetics (inherited and new variation) to alter neurodevelopmental, immune, oxidative stress and mitochondrial pathways. It is proposed that this influences development in affected individuals, leading to neurodevelopmental differences (disorders) such as autism. Postnatal environments may also contribute to the severity of symptoms (Siu & Weksberg, 2017).

Structural and functional brain imaging studies of ASD focused on the first years of life have identified neurological differences (see Wolff et al., 2018). These include increased cerebellar volume (grey and white matter) and atypical structural and functional connectivity. Research is ongoing to examine the relationship between neurology and cognitive and behaviour differences. Over time, hopefully, this will lead to a better understanding of the different subtypes of autism, leading to interventions that focus more specifically on supporting individuals' particular needs.

Environmental factors can be unsettling, as the discussion can result in parents (especially mothers) feeling blamed for their child's autism. Leo Kanner, who first described autism, noticed a lack of warmth from parents (particularly mothers). This led to the description of "refrigerator parenting" as a parenting style in the 1950s, which was **incorrectly** blamed for autism. However, there are known environmental factors which probably relate to the epigenetic factors described above.

---

**Environmental factors** associated with a diagnosis of autism:

- Neonatal hypoxia.
- Paternal age (>50, which increases the likelihood of a new genetic mutation).
- Maternal age (>40).
- Maternal obesity.
- Gestational diabetes.
- Time between pregnancies (a gap of fewer than 12 months increases the likelihood of autism).

- Medication during pregnancy (e.g. taking valproate, a medication used to manage seizure disorders).
- Folic acid supplementation may be protective (but too much may increase the risk of autism).
- Prematurity.                                                                        (Lord et al., 2020)

There is no doubt that this list is sobering. Many of the factors are beyond the control of parents. In isolation and in individual cases, the factors are not likely to be significant. Guilt, for example, about forgetting to take folic acid regularly or taking medication that may be essential to the parent but that could be associated with an increased risk of autism for the infant, or delaying parenthood until later in life, is entirely understandable but unhelpful and potentially distracting from the child and the family's current needs.

There is **no association** between autism and:

- Vaccination – although this continues to be a significant concern for some families.
- Hypertensive disease of pregnancy.
- Prolonged labour.
- Premature rupture of membranes.
- Birth by caesarean section or assisted vaginal delivery.
- Prenatal smoking.
- Assistive reproductive technology.                                                  (Lord et al., 2020)

In America, the *Diagnostic and Statistical Manual of Mental Disorders, Fifth Edition* (American Psychiatric Association, 2013) has specified the term "autism spectrum disorder." This terminology has been shared by the *International Classification of Diseases, 11th Revision* (World Health Organization, 2018), providing international agreement on language. Before the DSM-5, a range of terms had been used, often under the umbrella term "pervasive developmental disorder" (PDD). These included autism, autism spectrum disorder, autism spectrum condition, pathological demand avoidance, Asperger's syndrome and atypical autism. "Autistic features" was used for some children who did not fully meet the criteria for autism.

The writing of the DSM-5 criteria has simplified terminology but not the process of diagnosis or understanding the condition (see Chapter 2). "The autisms" is a recent description. As our knowledge of the causes and presentation of autism develops, it seems likely that, eventually, autism will be identified as a range of different conditions.

## Prevalence

The prevalence of autism in England is about 1 in 57 children (1.76%) (Roman-Urrestarazu et al., 2021). Data from children aged 5-19 years in state-funded education in England showed that more than four boys were diagnosed for every girl. This is within the ranges suggested in previous studies, but the question of undiagnosed girls with autism remains open. It seems likely that there are significant numbers of undiagnosed autistic girls.

The study also identified differences according to race/ethnicity, with the highest prevalence in children identified in the schools' census as black (2.11%) and the lowest in children identified in the schools' census as Roma/Irish traveller (0.85%).

## Girls

It is likely that the gender difference results from:

- Gender bias in screening, referral and diagnostic processes (these have been developed with boys in mind).
- Masking (camouflaging) so that autism may not be observed.
- Protective and/or compensatory factors (e.g. good organisational skills may compensate for some autistic differences).
- Different profiles of autistic girls/women that are not widely understood.
- Research often excludes girls (due to low numbers), perpetuating bias.

---

Gender differences also exist in communication

- Diagnostic criteria have been developed to identify the behavioural characteristics of autism. Girls may have more internalised autistic presentation so that their diagnosis is often later.
- Girls generally have better conversational reciprocity, language and pragmatics, and non-verbal communication skills than boys with autism (but weaker than neurotypical girls).
- Autistic girls may be chatty and sociable or shy and isolated.
- It is common for autistic girls to have a couple of strong friendships, but to find it more difficult to socialise in groups (although this difficulty may be masked effectively).

---

- They may feel an intense desire to fit in, but also a desire to express individuality (e.g. through hair, piercings, clothing choices) (Autistic Girls Network, 2022).
- Females are more likely than autistic males to be aware of difficulties with pragmatic, language and social behaviours (Sturrock et al., 2020).

## Useful resource

*Autism, Girls, & Keeping It All Inside* (Autistic Girls Network, 2022)

## Bilingualism

Bilingualism facilitates children and young people's participation in their families and within their communities, and enriches their lives. Autistic people must be provided with equal access and appropriate support for language learning. As with any child or young person, consider the child/young person's home language.

Digard and Davis' (2021) review summarises that bilingual autistic children do not have additional language difficulties as a result of their bilingualism. As is the case with other children, they can have smaller vocabularies early in childhood and mix languages, but this does not often persist. There is some evidence that learning two languages from a young age could help with perspective-taking (Digard & Davis, 2021).

## Useful resource

*Bilingualism in Autism: Evidence and Recommendations for Clinical Practice*, leaflets for clinician and families in several languages (Digard & Davis, 2021; available online)

*Working with Children Experiencing Speech and Language Disorders in a Bilingual Context* (Pert, 2022)

Diagnostic overshadowing may occur when other diagnoses are used to explain a young person's difficulties (e.g. eating disorder, ADHD, anxiety), which may result in delay or lack of appropriate autism diagnosis. Diagnostic overshadowing also occurs when the autism and/or any learning disability is accepted as the explanation for any physical or mental health concerns. This contributes to the stark statistics: "On average, males with a learning disability die 22 years younger than males from the general population, and females 26 years younger than females [from] the general population" (White et al., 2022).

## More autistic people?

There are currently more autistic people, and for some, diagnosis occurs at younger ages. The increase in numbers is real; the reason for this is not entirely straightforward. It seems clear that the diagnostic criteria have been increasingly flexible, but more people also need specialist support.

More reliable and broader definitions of autism have resulted in:

- Increased awareness of autism in schools and healthcare.
- More children are being diagnosed at a younger age, which increases the total number of people diagnosed with autism.
- More adults are being diagnosed and/or are self-identifying as autistic.
- Increased awareness as parents advocate for services, and some influential autistic adults and expert parents have communicated to large numbers through scientific publications (e.g. Temple Grandin).
- Media such as films (*Rain Man*), TV (BBC's *The A Word*), books, memoires and the internet, social media and podcasts (e.g. BBC Sounds' *1800 Seconds on Autism*) have increased awareness and requests for diagnosis.
- The concept of autism has broadened (classic autism → autism spectrum disorder → classic + other pervasive developmental disorders → PDDs not otherwise specified → autism).
- People with significant learning difficulties are now more likely to have their autism recognised and diagnosed.
- More women and girls are being diagnosed.
- The way that the number of people with autism is captured has changed.
- Autism is much more commonly used where there is also an identifiable medical disorder (conditions that are highly associated with autism, e.g. Fragile X syndrome) and autism is diagnosed alongside other diagnoses (e.g. Down syndrome and autism, ADHD and autism), where previously this would not have been the case.
- Autism is diagnosed more often in children and young people who do not have learning difficulties.
- The identification of autism in prevalence studies can be inconsistent, resulting in figures that may be considered unreliable (e.g. may include parent reports, inferring from school paperwork, self-diagnosis).

## Wellbeing

Dr Peter Vermeulen has written and spoken widely about autism and the pursuit of happiness (e.g. Vermeulen, 2019). Wellbeing and mental health have a higher profile than ever for all children and young people. Promoting emotional wellbeing, specifically autistic happiness, should be acknowledged in outcomes/success criteria for children and young people with autism, rather than relying on the traditional outcome measures (e.g. decreasing autism symptoms, employment, independence/support needs). As for anyone, the critical factor is identifying what is essential to the young person.

Families with a child with autism are extremely vulnerable to mental ill health. The shock of a diagnosis, even when expected, can be overwhelming. Appropriate early help is needed to support families to adapt to the news and develop support networks, including supporting the families to understand their children and maintain their wellbeing so they can engage with professionals working with them.

> The mother of ten-year-old Jay talked with his SLT about her response to her son's diagnosis seven years earlier: "I feel that the black cloud that appeared when he was diagnosed is just starting to lift."

Early and consistent support is critical to supporting the wellbeing and resilience of families with an autistic child.

## Protective factors

Some factors, such as executive function skills and resilience, may be protective for a person with autism to have a good quality of life. It is essential to consider this separately from masking or camouflaging, where the individual has learned (consciously or unconsciously) to hide their autism. This is likely to be harmful to the individual; masking comes at a very high cost to the person's mental health.

A good outcome, measured by the wellbeing of the autistic young person, may not look the same as for a young person without autism. The extent of language and learning difficulties might have an impact on this. The extent of mental ill health and suicide in young people with autism remains horrifying. The 2020 coronavirus pandemic significantly impacted young people's access to support networks and mental health services. Compared to the general public, autistic people in June and July 2020 were seven times more likely to be chronically lonely, and nine out of ten autistic people worried about their mental health during lockdown (National Autistic Society, 2020).

In *The Real Experts* (Sutton, 2015), adults with autism have written and spoken powerfully about their experiences of interventions as children and the negative impact of these on their sense of self and mental health. This reinforces the need to flexibly support children and young people, considering their needs in terms of the environment (and making appropriate changes to the environment to enable participation) and developing the skills of the people around them to provide effective support. "Neurodiversity is not against the idea of therapy and education for autism-related difficulties, as long as this therapy is geared toward improving quality of life and not toward eliminating non-normative differences" (p. 7) (Autistic Self Advocacy Network, 2015).

## Impact of autism

The impact of autism is hugely diverse and depends on the profile of the individual and their social context: the people with whom they spend time. Associated learning and language difficulties will affect the individual's experience. Those with more significant language and/or learning difficulties are often less able to share their experiences/self-advocate.

Much has been written about an autistic person's difficulties and differences. Identifying, acknowledging and using their strengths are vital. These may include (but are not limited to):

- High level of motivation for particular interests: skill, knowledge, vocabulary, persistence, engagement.
- Accuracy and reliability.
- Eye for detail.
- Memory for facts and figures.

> Stephen Wiltshire MBE is an architectural artist. He can look at a subject once and then draw a detailed picture, this includes drawing large, accurate city scenes after a single viewing, e.g. a 20-minute helicopter ride. He has a permanent gallery in London.
>
> Link to Stephen Wiltshire's website: www.stephenwiltshire.co.uk

- A different perspective that can result in remarkable insights.
- Empathy.

Temple Grandin is a professor of animal sciences, particularly renowned for her work on animals in abattoirs in the United States. Her ability to understand the animals, for example, their vocalisations and sensory preferences, has impacted animal handling, equipment, and plant design, resulting in more humane slaughter.

Link to Temple Grandin's website: www.templegrandin.com

- Creative talents.
- Honest and non-judgmental.
- Loyalty in social relationships.

The mother of Mark, a 15-year-old with autism and significant learning difficulties, thought about his strengths, including his love of screens and his fantastic eye for detail, and envisaged a future for him monitoring security cameras.

A person's interests are likely to make a difference in the impact of their autism: this can be positive and life-affirming, and results in opportunities (e.g. in mathematics, science, arts and business). There are many examples of successful autistic adults and suggestions of historical figures who may have been autistic.

Derek Paravicini is blind, has severe learning difficulties and is on the autism spectrum. He is a renowned, creative pianist with a repertoire of tens of thousands of pieces learned fast by listening. He performs across the United Kingdom and plays with his quartet and on his YouTube channel.

Link to Derek Paravicini's website: www.derekparaviciniquartet.com

## Summary

- Autism remains complex. Many differences can be identified, but differences do not automatically equate to need.
- Developing our appreciation and understanding of neurodiversity is essential to understanding individuals and society.
- The neurotypical society does not yet accommodate the needs of neurodivergent people; therefore, autism remains challenging for many children and young people.
- It is essential to develop our awareness and skills to support autistic children and young people.

# References

American Psychiatric Association, 2013. *Diagnostic and Statistical Manual of Mental Disorders (DSM-5)*. 5th ed. Washington, DC: American Psychiatric Publishing.

Autistic Girls Network, 2022. *Autism, Girls, & Keeping It All Inside*. [Online] Available at: https://autisticgirlsnetwork.org/wp-content/uploads/2022/03/Keeping-it-all-inside.pdf [Accessed 22 7 2022].

Autistic Self Advocacy Network, 2015. *A Curriculum for Self Advocates*. [Online] Available at: https://autisticadvocacy.org/wp-content/uploads/2015/02/CurriculumForSelfAdvocates_r7.pdf [Accessed 13 10 2022].

Coleman, M. & Gillberg, C., 2012. *The Autisms*. Oxford: Oxford University Press.

Cullen, R., 2021. *The Autistic Communication Hypothesis*. [Online] Available at: https://aucademy.co.uk/rachel-cullen-they-them/ [Accessed 15 08 2022].

Digard, B. G. & Davis, R., 2021. *Bilingualism in Autism: Evidence and Recommendations for Clinical Practice*. [Online] Available at: https://doi.org/10.31219/osf.io/uyzkg [Accessed 13 04 2022].

Fletcher-Watson, S. & Happé, F., 2019. *Autism: A New Introduction to Psychological Theory and Current Debate*. London: Routledge.

Girault, J. B. & Piven, J., 2020. The Neurodevelopment of Autism from Infancy Through Toddlerhood. *Neuroimaging Clinics of North America*, 30(1), pp. 97–114.

Hearst, C., 2022. *AutAngel – Resources*. [Online] Available at: https://www.autangel.org.uk/resources/ [Accessed 17 08 2022].

Lord, C. et al., 2020. Autism Spectrum Disorder. *Nature Reviews Disease Primers*, 6(5).

Milton, D., 2012. On the Ontological Status of Autism: The 'Double Empathy Problem'. *Disability and Society*, 27(6), pp. 883–887.

National Autistic Society, 2018. *Autism Facts and History*. [Online] Available at: www.autism.org.uk/about/what-is/myths-facts-stats.aspx [Accessed 23 08 2020].

National Autistic Society, 2020. *Left Stranded: The Impact of Coronavirus on Autistic People and Their Families in the UK*. London: National Autistic Society.

Ozonoff, S. et al., 2011. Recurrence Risk for Autism Spectrum Disorders: A Baby Siblings Research Consortium Study. *Pediatrics*, 128(3).

Pert, S., 2022. *Working with Children Experiencing Speech and Language Disorders in a Bilingual Context*. London: Routledge.

Prizant, B. M., 2019. *A Different Way of Seeing Autism: Uniquely Human*. London: Souvenir Press.

Roman-Urrestarazu, A. et al., 2021. Association of Race/Ethnicity and Social Disadvantage With Autism Prevalence in 7 Million School Children in England. *JAMAPediatrics*, 29(3), p. e210054.

Rose, K., 2022a. YouTube: An introduction to monotropism. https://www.youtube.com/watch?v=qUFDAevkd3E

Rose, K., 2022b. YouTube: An introduction to the double empathy problem. https://www.youtube.com/watch?v=qpXwYD9bGyU

Silberman, S., 2015. *Neurotribes*. London: Allen & Unwin.

Siu, M. T. & Weksberg, R., 2017. Epigenetics of Autism Spectrum. In: R. Delgado-Morales, ed. *Neuroepigenomics in Aging and Disease (Advances in Experimental Medicine and Biology)*. New York: Springer International Publishing.

Sturrock, A., Marsden, A., Adams, C. & Freed, J., 2020. Observational and Reported Measures of Language and Pragmatics in Young People with Autism: A Comparison of Respondent Data and Gender Profiles. *Journal of Autism and Developmental Disorders*, 50, pp. 812–30.

Sutton, M., ed., 2015. *The Real Experts: Readings for Parents of Autistic Children*. Fort Worth: Autonomous Press.

Vermeulen, P., 2019. *CRAE Annual Lecture*. London: CRAE.

Walker, N., 2015. What Is Autism?. In: M. Sutton, ed. *The Real Experts: Readings for Parents of Autistic Children*. Fort Worth: Autonomous Press, pp. 11–20.

White, A. et al., 2022. *Learning from the Lives and Deaths – People with a Learning Disability and Autistic People (LeDeR) Report for 2021 (LeDeR 2021)*. London: Autism and Learning Disability Partnership, King's College.

Wing, L., 1996. *The Autistic Spectrum: A Guide for Parents and Professionals*. London: Constable and Co.

Wiśniowiecka-Kowalnik, B. & Nowako, B. A., 2019. Genetics and Epigenetics of Autism Spectrum Disorder—Current. *Journal of Applied Genetics*, 60, pp. 37–47.

Wolff, J. J., Jacob, S. & Elison, J. T., 2018. The Journey to Autism: Insights from Neuroimaging Studies of Infants and Toddlers. *Development and Psychopathology*, 30, pp. 479–495.

World Health Organization, 2018. [Online] Available at: https://icd.who.int/browse11/l-m/en#/http://id.who.int/icd/entity/437815624 [Accessed 08 08 2020].

# DIAGNOSIS AND ASSOCIATED DIAGNOSES
# (EMBRACING COMPLEXITY)

DOI: 10.4324/9781003154334-3

**Key points**

Diagnosis can be a helpful signpost, but identification of strengths and needs is the priority.

**Focus on**

- Working as part of a team to support the child/young person and their family.
- Identifying strengths and needs.

# Introduction

Diagnosis can be a helpful signpost. In some parts of the United Kingdom, a diagnosis is no longer necessary to access appropriate support. However, individuals and their families still find a diagnosis beneficial and sometimes essential to find and access help. This is complex as autistic children and young people are not a homogeneous group: autism does not mean the same thing to everyone. A clear description of a young person's strengths and needs is most helpful.

# Background

Autism spectrum disorder (ASD) is a medical diagnosis within the group of neurodevelopmental disorders. In recent years, the diagnostic label has been simplified. Previously, an attempt was made to identify subgroups, including autistic disorder, Asperger's syndrome, atypical autism and pervasive development disorder – not otherwise specified (PDD-NOS). These different diagnostic groups were not homogeneous, making the diagnoses confusing for individuals, their families and professionals.

The term "spectrum" shows the heterogenicity of people with autism. "Constellation" is now sometimes used to reflect the multidimensional nature of autism. This has not yet reached the diagnostic process.

A diagnosis of ASD is based on the identification of "deficits" in social communication and repetitive patterns of interest/behaviour, but is widely discussed clinically as "differences." Many people prefer "autism spectrum" (which inadvertently confuses it with Asperger's syndrome when abbreviated: AS) or autism; these do not have the negative connotations of "disorder" nor the implication of disease requiring treatment.

## The path to a diagnosis

The path to a diagnosis is often slow, confusing and frustrating. "Children and young people with suspected autism wait too long before being provided with a diagnostic assessment" (NHS England, 2019).

This wait for a diagnosis can delay support and impact on developing positive working relationships between professionals and families. A rapid review in the United Kingdom looked at effective and safe ways to streamline the diagnostic process to make it faster and more efficient without losing quality (Abrahamson et al., 2020). This review identified theories which are now being tested relating to the diagnostic pathway, including "initial recognition of possible autism; referral and triaging; diagnostic model," and at all stages of the process: "working in partnership with families; interagency working; and training, service evaluation and development" (Abrahamson et al., 2021).

The UK's National Institute of Health and Care Excellence (NICE) specifies that an autism team should diagnose autism: a multidisciplinary team (MDT) composed of a paediatrician or child and adolescent psychiatrist, a clinical or educational psychologist and a speech and language therapist (SLT), working with the individual and their family (National Institute of Health and Care Excellence [NICE], 2017).

In the United Kingdom, there is increasing support for a more flexible diagnostic process, which can take account of the complexity of the presentation of many children so that assessment can reflect the young person's complexity.

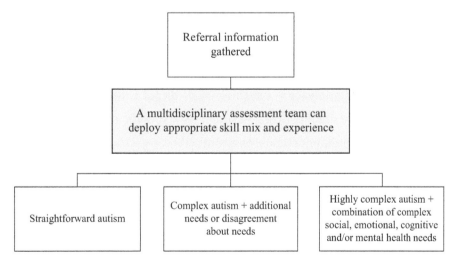

**FIGURE 2.1** Model for diagnostic pathway: embracing complexity.

Additional needs often accompany a diagnosis of autism so that autistic youngsters can accumulate several diagnoses (known within the medical model as "co-morbidities"). The Embracing Complexity Coalition (ECC, 2019a) highlights concerns about waiting times for diagnosis and inadequate recognition or planning for the likelihood of multiple neurodevelopmental diagnoses by health services. The coalition recommends that diagnostic pathways consider this, and proposes considering these potential diagnoses within one pathway rather than referring the child/young person to different pathways for different diagnostic questions. Some parts of the United Kingdom are implementing a more inclusive diagnostic process with neurodevelopment clinics rather than separate autism and attention deficit hyperactivity disorder (ADHD) clinics (ECC, 2019b).

## Role of SLTs

SLTs have a unique role in

- Identifying social and communication characteristics.
- Contributing to the differential diagnosis of autistic people.
- Identifying co-morbidities.
- Delivering therapy.
- Training people looking after/educating autistic people. (Royal College of Speech and Language Therapists, n.d.)

All SLTs working with children and young people have a role in identifying possible autism. Chapter 1 includes a list of behaviours that may be observed, focusing on differences in communication, interests and information processing, and sensory differences. This can help identify and describe children and young people who should be referred for diagnostic assessment (see section titled "Possible indicators") using the local route: referral to a paediatrician or child and adolescent psychiatrist or direct referral to a diagnostic team. Some specialist SLTs have diagnostic assessment as a specific part of their role. See section titled "Role of SLTs in diagnostic assessment."

Autistic children may or may not have difficulties expressing themselves verbally, but they will have communication differences. Most very young neurotypical children can communicate proficiently before they can express themselves verbally (see section titled "Typical early communication").

When there is concern about a child's development, identifying strengths and needs requires:

- Observation.
- Discussion with:
  - Parent/carer.
  - Educational setting.

This provides information for the diagnostic team to help differentiate between language delay/disorder (the youngster usually uses alternative/supplementary strategies) and autism (use of alternative/supplementary strategies will be limited or idiosyncratic) and other needs. A child with a language delay/disorder will likely use many of the typical early communication strategies to communicate, despite their lack of spoken language. They may make their feelings known very clearly using eye gaze, facial expression and body language, and use and respond to a pointing gesture (if this is culturally appropriate) from around 12 months. An autistic child will be less sophisticated in coordinating their non-verbal strategies.

---

**TYPICAL EARLY COMMUNICATION**

In a typically developing child, we might expect to see an infant:

- <u>Looking towards</u> **showing interest.**
- <u>Leaning out of carer's arms</u> when they want **to get away.**
- <u>Reaching up</u> to be **carried.**
- <u>Turning towards</u> a favourite person, **demonstrating preference.**
- <u>Turning the body away</u> or <u>hiding behind</u> to **avoid interaction.**
- <u>Waving</u> **to greet/say bye.**
- <u>Peeping</u> to **initiate/sustain interaction.**
- <u>Looking to a person and object</u> to **share an interest.**
- <u>Reaching</u> to **request.**
- <u>Pointing and looking to the person</u> to **request** or **show** item out of reach.
- <u>Giving</u> an item to an adult to **share interest/show, ask for an explanation or request help.**

A single word can express many meanings using prosody, body language and facial expression. For example, "Car" – I want to go in the car. It's a car. I've had enough, and I want to leave now! I like the car. Is it a car? Give me the (toy) car. Can we go in the car? I'm not getting in the car! Fast car. New car.

---

Some TV shows have obvious examples of effective pre-verbal and non-verbal communication, e.g. Timmy Time, Bing, In the Night Garden, Teletubbies and The Clangers.

The presence or absence of some of these features may result from different social expectations within a family. For example, in some communities, it is not socially appropriate to point, but a typically developing infant would follow their mother's eye gaze to look at an interesting object.

Some behaviours are more likely to be seen in an autistic youngster. When these occur, professionals need to be particularly vigilant, but they are not diagnostic on their own. The absence of these does not exclude autism.

**POSSIBLE INDICATORS**

Social communication:

- Limited use of conventional gestures, e.g. pointing, waving, showing or pretending (e.g. miming sipping from a cup).
- No or delayed speech, with no or limited attempt to compensate (e.g. through gesture).
- Little imitation or pretend in play.
- **Regression in language skills** (e.g. stopping using previously established words).
- Using another person's hand as a tool.
- Not appearing to share excitement/joy.
- Not responding to own name.
- Not appearing to share interests or activities with others.
- Limited or unusual eye gaze.
- Unusual prosody/accent.
- Lack of speech sounds.
- Echolalia: repeating the final word may be typical, but intonation is a clue. The imitation of an adult's questioning tone is echolalic rather than communicative.

Behaviours and interests:

- Rituals, e.g. lining up toys repeatedly.
- Intense focus on unusual items (switches, boingy doorstoppers, washing machine, wheels).

- Focus on particular interests to the exclusion of other interests and activities.
- Difficulty coordinating verbal and non-verbal communication.

Motor and sensory:

- Unusual finger, hand or body movements, might include finger posturing, hand flapping or toe walking.
- Unusual sensory interests/skills (sniffing objects to identify ownership, spotting detail within a complex situation, looking in a particular way, e.g. using peripheral vision).
- Under and/or over-responsive to sensory information. For example, seeking or avoiding messy play and/or limited eating – with very strong sensory preferences: texture, temperature, colour and brand. May be highly skilled at detecting changes from their preferred food, might cover ears, spin on a swing, chew on items, e.g. clothing, pencils. Different awareness of bodily functions which might impact toileting, appetite, response to pain and/or awareness of emotions.

Emotional regulation:

- Reliant on others to calm.
- Unable to calm with support from others.
- Extreme anxiety.

Very early indicators:

- Eye gaze: unusual quality or not looking at people's faces.
- Lack of babbling and/or babbling "conversations" with a caregiver.
- Limited use of gestures (e.g. waving).
- Limited use of vocalisation (e.g. "oops," "uh-oh").
- No response to name; appears deaf at times.
- No smile.

These indicators may immediately raise concerns about neurodevelopmental differences/disorders, including autism. Different biological and cognitive differences (including autism, a sensory impairment, developmental delay, deafness and motor difficulties) may cause these behaviours. Neurotypical children may show behaviours that appear autistic.

> For example, infants can hold their hands and look at them intently; many young children will flap their hands when excited; adult lottery winners shown on TV jump and vocalise loudly; and some children will toe walk or be highly focused on a repetitive activity.

Individually, none of these is indicative of autism. However, this deserves attention where the pattern and the intensity of the differences are substantial, particularly where the differences impact the child's interaction.

> Lee's focus on the washing machine was so intense that it was difficult to engage him in another activity.

Where these indicators are reported or observed, it is helpful to broadly consider the child or young person's strengths and needs. For a youngster referred to speech and language therapy, consider onward referral and discuss with their parent/carer.

## Speech and language therapy information when a diagnosis may be initiated

When indicators appear for a child or young person known to speech and language therapy, or there is a discussion about the possibility of autism, it is essential to be proactive. Usual assessment is relevant: notice, gather and record observations that could help understand the child's speech, language and communication strengths and needs. When autism is a possibility, it can be beneficial to consider and document the areas focused on within the autism diagnostic criteria:

- "Persistent deficits in initiating and sustaining social communication and reciprocal social interactions."
- "Persistent restricted, repetitive, and inflexible patterns of behaviour, interests, or activities." (World Health Organization, 2022)

Consider:

- <u>What</u> the child/young person is communicating. Look for lots of different reasons for communication expressed through any means.
- <u>How</u> they are communicating. Are they using conventional means and/or more idiosyncratic? How are the different means coordinated?

**TABLE 2.1** Communication: means and reasons

| | | Reasons: |
|---|---|---|
| pre-intentional | Self-injury/hurting | |
| | Escape | |
| | Crying/screaming | |
| | Proximity | |
| | Touch (hug) | |
| | Reach | |
| ↓ | Push | |
| intentional | Give | |
| | Take hand | |
| | Wave | |
| | Point (contact/distant) | |
| ↓ | Nod/shake head | |
| conventional | Facial expression | |
| | Eye gaze | |
| | Vocalisation | |
| | Object | |
| | Symbol | |
| ↓ | Sign | |
| Symbolic | Speech<br>• Intonation<br>• Style<br>• Vocabulary | |
| | Join words (speech/signs/symbols) | |
| Exploratory/sensory play (bubbles, children's soapy foam, a balloon/pump and a noisy pig) | | |
| Cause and effect play (pop-up/wind-up toys, car/ball runs, spinner/whirler) | | |
| Pretend play (doll/action figure, food, accessories) | | |
| Puzzle (inset puzzle, 3D construction puzzle, copying simple patterns with blocks. What if a piece is missing?) | | |
| Book (fiction, non-fiction, emotions, retelling) | | |
| Paper and pencils | | |
| Understanding:<br>Blank level <1, 1, 2, 3, 4<br>What helps: e.g. context, body language, tone of voice, social context, processing time | | |

*Name _____ Date _____*

Consider whether speech, language and communication skills are

- Delayed (following a typical developmental sequence but at a slower rate) and likely to catch up.
- Disordered (following an unusual developmental sequence or pattern), e.g. autism with language disorder.
- As expected for age/in advance of their chronological age and/or other communication skills.

Autistic children and young people often have a "spiky" profile and may not follow a typical developmental path. A relative strength (e.g. saying a few words) may mask difficulty with another aspect (e.g. being able to express a range of meanings). While some children may be able to express a range of purposes using various means, there may be significant difficulty in coordinating these: using language, intonation, facial expression and eye gaze together to express meaning or interpret another person's communication.

---

Lara greets familiar adults by name with a beaming smile, usually followed up with a compliment about the person's appearance, e.g. "I like your nails." However, her understanding is extremely limited, and she cannot follow this up with further conversation or answer a follow-up question.

---

Poppy's language skills were as expected for her age. She was able to use eye gaze, facial expression and body language, but the quality of her interaction was rather learned. She had an unexpected accent for her family but not for her region. She frequently misunderstood the subtle social complexities of teenage life, leading to difficult social situations: arguments with friends and trouble at school for breaking unspoken rules. When finally diagnosed with autism, Poppy, her family and her school could understand and accommodate her communication strengths and needs.

---

## School-aged children and young people

Sometimes concern about social communication and possible autism arises later. If this is the case, the young person's language skills may appear to follow a more typical developmental pattern, so they spontaneously use verbal language for various purposes. Concerns may be identified for a variety of reasons that might include (but are not limited to):

- Social difficulties.
- Behaviours of concern.
- Intensity of interests.

- Idiosyncratic communication.
- Emotional difficulties.

Some children and young people may present with apparently different concerns (e.g. an eating disorder), but further investigation may elicit broader concerns about social communication. Some young people (including girls) are particularly vulnerable to missing an autism diagnosis. This can be because their needs may be more subtle, they may use significant energy in masking (camouflaging) their differences and their special interests might be considered typical for their age. However, a closer investigation may elicit information about the unusual intensity and focus of their interest. They may not present with difficulties to services, or concerns may be raised about the young person.

Concerns may be raised by

- Young person.
- Parents/carers.
- School.
- Or as a result of involvement with other services: a youth offending team, child and adolescent mental health services, GP, school nurse, gender identity clinic, other universal health professionals (e.g. dentist) or professionals seen for another reason (e.g. differences noted by a paediatrician when a child is seen for an acute medical issue, or a physio seeing a child for toe walking), but the presentation may not initially suggest autism as a possibility.

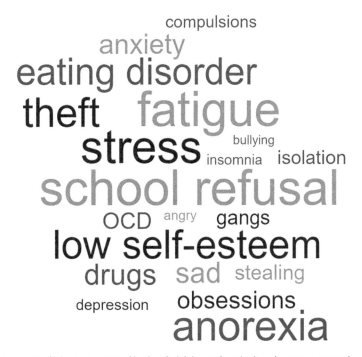

FIGURE 2.2 Some possible concerns that might be raised about young people.

These concerns may then be reported through different systems. In the United Kingdom, a local diagnostic pathway for neurodevelopmental conditions or an autism pathway exists, which will (eventually) assess the child/young person's strengths and needs and diagnose as appropriate. Information about early development is beneficial (e.g. in England, there may be relevant information in the child's personal health record, their "red book" → eredbook).

As with younger children, a range of information is relevant. Differences may be subtle and only easily evident in some settings as the young person may be proficient at masking. However, the cost to energy and wellbeing will be evident.

Mark was a bright nine-year-old attending his local primary school. His school was not concerned about his progress academically or socially, but his mother was persistent in her insistence that he was struggling. Mark was often agitated when he returned home from school and frequently had tantrums for apparently little reasons at home. His teacher was initially unconcerned about Mark's social interaction, as she was not aware of any issues in school. It was helpful to identify specific examples of ambiguous language that he had difficulty understanding in "live" social settings, despite good understanding in situations where he was not involved (e.g. in his reading or when watching as an outsider). In school, he masked these difficulties, but once home in an unguarded, familiar situation with people he knew he understood and could trust, Mark expressed the anxiety and frustration he experienced, often dramatically. Everyone listening to each other's perspectives meant that all were able to acknowledge his strengths and needs, leading to more effective learning in school with discrete social support and calmer afternoons at home.

Mark and his family embraced his diagnosis, and it helped the school accommodate his subtle but significant needs. Knowing he was autistic helped him to negotiate the world effectively while maintaining his skills and interests in his unique way.

**Special interests** may be unusual and obvious (e.g. vacuum cleaners, boingy doorstops). For some autistic children and young people, their interests may appear appropriate so they may be dismissed. This is particularly true for girls who may be appropriately interested in horses, make-up, music icons or fashion. However, the intensity and focus, along with the lack of flexibility, may be more than would be expected and enough to fulfil the diagnostic criteria, e.g. ICD-11: "Persistent preoccupation with one or more special interests, parts of objects, or specific types of stimuli (including media)" (World Health Organization, 2022).

Sarah loved horses. She read about horses, played horses with friends at break-time, had horse toys and played imaginatively with them. Initially, this interest was dismissed in considering referral to the autism team, and her friendships and play were evidence of her sociability and imagination. However, as she got older and had consistent friendship difficulties, which impacted her wellbeing and learning, her interest's persistence, intensity and inflexibility were acknowledged as unusual, and she was referred to the autism team. Following her diagnosis, she continued to love horses and went on to get work experience in a local stable. Sarah and her love of horses were welcomed enthusiastically, and her wealth of (sometimes idiosyncratic) knowledge made her an asset to the team.

## Talking with families about referral

Careful discussion with the family about their understanding of their child's needs is essential alongside referral. When parents/carers arrive at a diagnostic clinic unaware of the appointment's purpose and without having the opportunity to talk about their child's needs, it can become extremely difficult for both family and professionals. Sometimes they have not heard of autism, which can be highly distressing and challenging for everyone.

Outline of a possible script for talking with parent/carer before referral to the diagnostic team:

"We've talked about your child's speaking and listening skills. These are different to other children of their age (give detail relevant to the individual).

I've noticed that *Sam* is very interested in..., and they are helped by... (use information observed and that provided by parent/carer).

*Sam* does have some social (communication) difficulties, e.g....

We sometimes see this in a child with autism. I want to refer *Sam* to the social communication/autism (use local term) team. They will be able to learn more about *Sam*'s communication skills and behaviour. They will work with you (and the school/nursery) to find out about your child's strengths and needs, whether or not *Sam* has autism or other social communication needs and what support might be needed.

Have you heard of autism? Thought about it?

What do you think?"

It is helpful to provide this information in writing at the time of the appointment with contact details for queries.

## Referral

The NICE guidelines provide clear information about referral to an autism team for diagnostic assessment. Any SLT who has had contact with the child will be able to give helpful information in the form of a speech, language and communication profile about the child within the context of their contacts: assessment and response to intervention.

Discussion of children with complex or ambiguous needs in supervision is essential. It may be appropriate to defer referral to the autism team, for example, when concerns are insufficient or when parents/carers decline a referral. When this is the case, document the discussion, provide support for the needs identified and arrange a review when the referral can be revisited.

## What to do

*Observation*

Whether or not the referral to speech and language therapy is for diagnostic assessment, a priority is the identification of the child/young person's strengths and needs. Observation in a setting familiar to the child/young person provides naturalistic information about their communication and participation (see Chapter 3).

*Assessment*

Specialist assessments, such as the Autism Diagnostic Observation Schedule (ADOS-2) (Lord et al., 2012), are designed to support a diagnosis of autism. However, these typically require training to administer, are very strict in structure and objects used, are not screening tools and would not be appropriate or practical to use outside a diagnostic setting. Any therapist can use activities to attempt to elicit responses from a child or young person. Learning about a young person's interests and then using these within the assessment is likely to support participation. Discussion with parents/carers about their observations of the child/young person and how they might be similar or different to siblings or other children in the community will provide helpful information.

As part of an assessment that might be used to inform a diagnosis and to identify strengths and needs, but not specifically diagnostic, it is helpful to have activities that are likely to be motivating to probe skills and needs.

Consider providing <u>visual support</u>. Many children benefit from knowing what is happening when they see an unfamiliar person; supporting this visually is helpful. This could be a list written down or drawn to tick off or a more traditional timetable with symbols (do2learn.com has free symbols if commercial symbol software is unavailable). Notice:

- Is this useful?
- Does the child look at it?
- Engage with the content?

Be aware that scaffolding may enable participation and mask difficulties that could be evident without support.

- Exploratory/sensory play activities are engaging for lots of children and young people. For example, use bubbles, children's soapy foam, a balloon/pump and a noisy pig. Have fun! Keep these out of reach, so the child can access the play and fun but manage access to the resource. This increases opportunities for any communication (including non-verbal).
- Cause and effect play ideas: pop-up/wind-up toys, car/ball runs, spinner/whirler.
- Pretend play: doll/action figure (Spiderman or similar!), food, accessories.
- Puzzle: inset puzzle, 3D construction puzzle, copying simple patterns (photo or photocopied patterns) with blocks. What if a piece is missing (consider "accidentally" leaving a part in the box/bag)?
- Book: having books with few words but a variety of interests, including non-fiction and people, to provide an opportunity to talk about what other people might say and think and their emotions.
- Paper and pencils or whiteboard/markers (see Table 2.1, p. 33).

Remember, you are looking for communication: purposeful, conventional and incidental. Notice, does the youngster:

- Watch as you play?
- Request (reach, grab, vocalise, point)?
- Share an interest, looking at you/carer?
- Look between the item and you?
- Anticipate (ready, steady...)?
- Protest/reject (wipe wet or foamy hands, vocalise, push item away, withdraw)?
- Show emotion: facial expression, motor mannerisms, body language?
- Show any indication of requesting help? how?

## Role of SLTs in diagnostic assessment

The NICE guidelines specify that an SLT is a core part of the autism team alongside a paediatrician or child and adolescent psychiatrist and a clinical or educational psychologist (National Institute of Health and Care Excellence [NICE], 2017). The Royal College of Speech and Language Therapists' (RCSLT) guidance (Royal College of Speech and Language Therapists, n.d.) reiterates that SLTs should be integral members of the diagnostic teams with a particular role in a differential diagnosis, e.g. autism, developmental language disorder (DLD) or language disorder with autism.

As part of the diagnostic team, the therapist assesses speech, language and communication using formal and informal means. Several well-established assessments and interview schedules are widely used within the diagnostic process. For example, the Autism Diagnostic Observation Schedule (ADOS-2) (Lord et al., 2012) and the Autism Diagnostic Interview, Revised (ADI-R) (Rutter et al., 2003) are regarded as "gold standard" tools to support diagnosis. The ADOS-2 standardised assessment uses semi-structured tasks to assess communication, social interaction, play and restricted and repetitive behaviours. Administration and scoring are highly standardised, and training is required. An SLT, with colleagues from the team, can use the ADOS-2 following this training.

## Diagnostic criteria

*The International Classification of Diseases, Eleventh Revision* (World Health Organization, 2022), known as ICD-11 and the *Diagnostic and Statistical Manual of Mental Disorders, 5th edition* (DSM-5) criteria (American Psychiatric Association, 2013) are widely used in the United Kingdom. Although they share some terminology, they are not identical. They share a focus on deficits in social communication and interaction and restricted, repetitive behaviour. They helpfully highlight sensory differences as a possible restricted or repetitive behaviour.

The ICD-11 (World Health Organization, 2022) is a system for coding medical diagnoses, diseases, signs and symptoms. It classifies autism spectrum disorder in the neurodevelopmental disorders category within the mental, behavioural or neurodevelopmental disorders section. It allows for the specification of intellectual development and functional language within the diagnosis. Full criteria can be found at https://icd.who.int/, which is regularly updated.

The DSM-5 (American Psychiatric Association, 2013) is a tool for categorising and diagnosing mental disorders. Full criteria can be found at www.autismspeaks.org/autism-diagnosis-criteria-dsm-5.

## Following diagnosis

A diagnosis of autism has a different meaning for each person. Some parents are relieved, having fought and waited for an assessment and can appear exultant. They have (finally) been listened to, and their concerns acknowledged and validated. More often, there is sadness. Sometimes, the response is surprise, confusion or denial. Even when it is expected, the long-term impact of the diagnosis can be profound. The task for the parent(s)/carer of sharing this diagnosis with the wider family can be difficult and exhausting.

Going to a doctor for an assessment and discussing "deficits", "impairments" and diagnosis imply disease. This suggests the need to look for a "cure," which can be some parents' immediate response. This approach is unhelpful. Many autistic people who have talked or written about their experiences consider that autism is a fundamental part of their person and that any approach attempting to treat it is problematic. However, for parents facing a new diagnosis, it is understandable that searching for treatments and a cure may be the initial and overwhelming response. Adequate family support is critical through the diagnosis (whatever the outcome) and beyond. Ensuring that the assessment culminates in identifying strengths, needs and effective support is crucial. It is vital that parents/carers feel trust in the professionals who are working with them and that they all work together. While professionals may be the autism experts, the parents/carers/family live with their own experience and have expert knowledge of their child and family.

The value of an assessment is the learning of the family so that they can better understand and advocate for their child (Lord, 2014). The final diagnosis may not be the most important aspect of the assessment. It is essential to clearly understand the strengths and needs of the child or young person and what support is likely to help. It should provide the family (including the child) with a plan of what is to come. This will include post-diagnostic support available locally (and beyond) from health, voluntary, education and social care. Identify a key worker (or a named person) to contact with queries and concerns.

After the diagnostic assessment, a profile of strengths and needs is a powerful tool.

**TABLE 2.2** Extract from a strengths and needs profile

| | What | Provision/support |
|---|---|---|
| Strengths | Music and dance<br><br>Zayn is a talented singer, and he enjoys writing lyrics and performing. He loves to dance and uses dance effectively to provide himself with breaks when anxious or agitated. | Opportunities to listen to music/dance daily, build into timetable in the setting, ensure opportunities to build on this in selecting options/leisure.<br><br>With Zayn, identify further opportunities to use music and dance to support across the week.<br><br>Use interest to support focus in other settings (consider background music, incorporate it into learning opportunities and celebrate this: writing song lyrics, performing). |
| | Language<br><br>Zayn uses spoken language to express himself (Blank level 3). He reads and writes, and this helps when agitated. | Use Zayn's good reading and writing to support spoken language. Check with him: what will help? |
| Needs | Zayn would like to have friends<br><br>Emotional regulation: behaviours of concern (damaging property, hurting self/others).<br><br>Zayn's good speaking skills mean that people can have unreasonably high expectations of his communication skills. | Develop secure, trusting relationships with adults in the setting. The adult is to be led by the young person. Spend time getting to know the young person's preferences and interests. Join in on their terms at their pace. Aim to understand from Zayn's point of view. **Trust and Zayn feeling safe are the foundation of any learning/skill development that can take place.**<br><br>Consider opportunities to develop relationships with peers. Use interests (e.g. music). Consider environment (copes better in a slightly busy but reasonably calm, predictable setting with a familiar adult nearby for reassurance).<br><br>Support from the autism team:<br><br>• Work with Zayn's community with mutual misunderstanding (double empathy problem).<br>  ○ Use less language.<br>  ○ Time to process.<br>  ○ Demonstrate.<br>  ○ Discretely check his understanding.<br>  ○ Say what you mean.<br>  ○ Write it down.<br>  ○ Carefully explore misunderstandings (not while he is agitated).<br>• Zayn's perspective-taking, looking at photos and videos using comic strips, consider analysing events that have happened using comic strips to support considering alternative perspectives (for all).<br>• Analysis of the function of behaviour: ?escape.<br>• Explore: what does "having friends" mean to Zayn? Who are his peers? |

## Differential diagnosis and co-occurring conditions

While this book is not designed for therapists working in highly specialised roles, it is helpful to have some awareness of the complexities of a differential diagnosis and co-occurring conditions. The NICE guidelines (National Institute of Health and Care Excellence [NICE], 2017) and diagnostic criteria provide helpful information where there are concerns about possible autism, including tricky diagnostic issues:

- Masking/camouflaging: some children and young people **mask** signs and symptoms of autism. This may be associated with effective coping mechanisms and/or a supportive environment. However, masking is often a protective mechanism that is unhelpful and harmful for the individual as they struggle to cope with an environment that is not supportive of neurodivergence. Masking may not be conscious and can be highly detrimental to wellbeing. It is particularly observed in children and young people with good language skills and autistic girls/women. As a result, they may be underdiagnosed.
- The possibility of autism may be overlooked for children and young people:
  - With **learning difficulties.**
  - With **English as an additional language.**
  - With **sensory impairments.**
- Children and young people in the **criminal justice system** are known to have a much higher rate of speech, language and communication needs than the general population, Bryan et al. (2007) found that up to 90% of young offenders have low language skills, with 46–67% of these in the poor or very poor range. Information about early development may not be easy to access for these young people, and undiagnosed autism is a possibility. Half of those entering the criminal justice system could be expected to have a neurodivergent condition (Criminal Justice Joint Inspection, 2021).

Autism **cannot be excluded** by:

- Good eye contact.
- Demonstrating affection for family members.
- Early hearing difficulties.
- Cultural differences and/or where English is not the family's first language. It is essential to consider the child's proficiency (understanding and expression) in their home language and their experience of life events and play. For example, not everyone celebrates birthdays, and celebrations do not always involve cakes with candles, so caution is needed in relying on a play activity based on unfamiliar experiences within an assessment; check with the family. Considering the young person's progress compared to

expected development within their community will support understanding cultural differences (e.g. in pointing and eye gaze) versus communication differences/difficulties.

- Children with a tricky start to life (e.g. adverse childhood experiences, looked after children and those living with parental mental or physical illness) are more complex to diagnose. For some children, information about early development may not be available.

Signs and symptoms of possible autism are not always recognised. Lack of agreement on the presentation of a child in different settings can be very challenging for all concerned. For example, parents may feel criticised, blamed and disempowered when they hear that their child is "fine at school," even when this is presented in a very positive light. This may be particularly difficult when the school attempts to support by sharing strategies, e.g. where a child is very passive (or shutdown) in school, which may be a coping response to a very challenging situation. The child has contained their anxiety all day, which is released within the familiarity of home.

## Differential diagnosis

A differential diagnosis is challenging, which is why a team approach is vital. There are many possible alternative diagnoses and co-occurring conditions. See section titled "Diagnostic criteria" and the NICE guidance (National Institute for Health and Care Excellence, 2020). Some are described as follows:

- **Developmental language disorder (DLD):** a child or young person with DLD but without autism will have typical imagination and play skills, relative strengths in social interaction with friendships (although communication difficulties may hinder these), and the young person will compensate for language difficulties with relatively good non-verbal communication skills.
  Where a language disorder occurs with autism, "language disorder with autism" can be diagnosed, and DLD would not be used (Bishop et al., 2017).
- **Learning disability:** a child or young person with a learning disability/difficulty without autism is likely to have a delay across all areas of development, and social communication and interests will be consistent with other areas.
  A learning disability can occur with autism, where there will be a relative weakness in social communication and interests compared to other areas. English school census data from 2017 suggests that this was identified in 18% of autistic children and young people (Roman-Urrestarazu et al., 2021), but this may be an underestimate as diagnostic overshadowing may mean that their learning difficulties are not identified. Autistica

states that "around 4 in 10 autistic people have a learning disability" (Autistica, n.d. c). Autism can be associated with learning difficulties.

- **Attention deficit hyperactivity disorder (ADHD)**: the child/young person is inattentive, impulsive and may be hyperactive, but when autism is not present, they will have appropriate non-verbal communication, social reciprocity and social understanding.

  A dual diagnosis of autism and ADHD is common: around 38% of autistic children also have ADHD (Rong et al., 2021). The presence of both diagnoses exacerbates the difficulties of the single diagnosis. A UK group of professional experts produced guidance for the diagnosis and treatment of co-occurring autism and ADHD: "Guidance for identification and treatment of individuals with attention deficit/hyperactivity disorder and autism spectrum disorder based upon expert consensus" (Young et al., 2020).

- **Developmental coordination disorder** (DCD), previously known as dyspraxia: a child with DCD will have difficulties with motor planning and organisation with typically developing play and language skills.

  Autistic children and young people often have motor difficulties to some extent. A recent review identified that up to 87% of the autistic population is affected by motor challenges (Zampella et al., 2021), although (at present) this is not recognised in the diagnostic criteria. DCD can occur with autism.

- **Ehlers-Danlos syndrome**/hypermobility spectrum disorders. In a Swedish retrospective study the rate of autism was about twice the expected rate (Kindgren et al., 2021).

- **Stereotypic movement disorder** (e.g. Tourette's syndrome): stereotyped or repetitive motor movements are seen in children and young people with autism, so this diagnosis would not be used in addition to autism. If the behaviour causes injuries, then an additional diagnosis may be given.

- **Mood disorder** (e.g. depression): in the absence of autism, the young person would have a history of typical social behaviour when not depressed or severely anxious (National Institute for Health and Care Excellence, 2020). Depression is more common in autistic adolescents and young adults, so more than half of autistic adults have had depression (Autistica, n.d. b). Diagnosis could be missed; while non-verbal communication (e.g. reduction in facial expression, less use of body language) is not diagnostic, it helps express mood. A flat affect may be attributed to the person's autism rather than exploring the possibility of a mood disorder: diagnostic overshadowing.

- **Anxiety disorder**: anxiety is frequently associated with autism – 42% of autistic children have an anxiety disorder compared to 3% of children who do not have autism (Autistica, n.d. a). It may be pronounced and a major presenting concern or internalised so that it is not evident to other people but at a high cost to the individual's energy and resilience.

- **Attachment disorder**: in the absence of autism, the youngster would usually have typical imaginative play and not demonstrate interests of unusual intensity. Within a nurturing environment they would usually progress well (National Institute for Health and Care Excellence, 2020). Attachment in autism may appear less secure as social interest may be expressed differently, impacting interactions with others. The Coventry Grid (Moran, 2010) highlights similarities in the presentation of children with autism and those with attachment difficulties and helpfully describes the typical differences between youngsters with autism and those with attachment difficulties. In the simplest terms, autistic children and young people tend to have a strongly cognitive approach to the world. In contrast, those with attachment difficulties have an intensely emotional approach to the world. A child with autism may experience attachment problems, and autism and an attachment disorder may be present.

- **Oppositional defiant disorder** (ODD) and **conduct disorder**: a child or young person persists with undesirable or unacceptable behaviour despite understanding that it is undesirable, no repetitive behaviour or interests and social interaction skills are otherwise adequate. In conduct disorder, the child or young person can use sophisticated strategies to avoid detection. These can be diagnosed in a child or young person with autism, but this is not common (although if other people are not seeing their perspective, they may appear oppositional). They are more likely to be diagnosed in a child with ADHD.

- **Obsessive-compulsive disorder** (OCD): onset is after early childhood and usually results in distress. The content of obsessions and rituals may be associated with avoiding harm. Repetitive behaviours can <u>appear</u> the same in autism and OCD, but in autism the behaviours reduce stress, while in OCD, the behaviours are stressful (Santorer et al., 2020). Autism may be undiagnosed in an adult with OCD (Wikramanayake et al., 2018).
  - ○ **Paediatric acute onset neuropsychiatric syndrome** (PANS): sudden onset of OCD or eating disorders in childhood; where this is associated with a specific infection it is known as PANDAS.

- **Schizophrenia**: usually develops after puberty. Hallucinations and/or delusions are symptoms.

- **Rett syndrome**: a rare genetic, neurological and developmental disorder that mainly affects girls and causes progressive loss of motor skills and language (characteristic "hand-wringing" movements). Does not co-occur with autism (World Health Organization, 2022).

- **Landau-Kleffner syndrome**: a rare epilepsy that occurs in children between three and nine years, characterised by loss of language skills and may be associated with difficulties with behaviour, social interaction, motor skills and learning.

- **Gender dysphoria** (DSM-5) or **gender incongruence** (ICD-11): a systematic review of the literature identified a link between autism spectrum disorder and gender dysphoria or gender incongruence (Kallitsounaki & Williams, 2022).

## Other conditions

- Severe hearing impairment: non-verbal communication, play, imagination, social interest and initiation of peer interaction are usually unaffected.
- Severe visual impairment: congenitally blind children may have some behaviours that overlap with autism, including repetitive finger or hand movements, no pointing, limited facial expressions, noise sensitivity, repetitive interests and parental reports of difficulty with imaginative play and/or establishing friendships (Williams et al., 2013).
- Selective mutism: consistent failure to speak in situations where there is an expectation of talking, despite speaking in other situations (usually home). There is an association between selective mutism and autism, and an assessment of children who communicate selectively should consider the possibility of autism (Steffenburg et al., 2018).
- Child abuse/maltreatment/trauma: children and young people who have experienced trauma or abuse can present with a marked change in behaviour associated with their experience.

Children and young people with other conditions can have a profile with difficulties that may have similarities with autism and may have a dual diagnosis, for example Down syndrome, Williams syndrome, Prader–Willi syndrome, Angelman syndrome and Fragile X.

## Pathological demand avoidance (PDA)

Avoiding demands is a typical response to anxiety. Demand avoidance is pathological for a youngster with PDA: it is so severe and pervasive that it interferes with everyday demands. PDA is a descriptive term introduced in the 1980s by Elizabeth Newson (professor of psychology at the University of Nottingham). However, it is controversial as critics claim it pathologises autistic people asserting their own needs or preferences or failing to acknowledge their self-advocacy (Milton, 2013).

PDA is not recognised in the DSM-5 or ICD-11 diagnostic criteria. It is usually accepted as being within the autism spectrum. However, the usual strategies for autistic children and young people are often not helpful for children and young people with a PDA profile.

The child or young person may:

- Resist/avoid the ordinary demands of life.
- Often use social strategies to distract, excuse, procrastinate or control.
- Appear superficially sociable (e.g. may have good language skills, able to use language for a range of purposes, interact effectively with people at times), but this **masks** subtle differences with social communication/interaction.

- Have difficulties with emotional regulation (e.g. extremes of moods).
- Escape into fantasy/imaginative play.
- Have an intense focus (may be on particular person/people).
- Have a great need for control: refuse, escape/leave the situation, withdraw or shut down.

Typical strategies to support an autistic child or young person are often ineffective. They tend to benefit from a flexible, non-confrontational and highly personalised approach that allows the young person to maintain control.

- Develop the relationship.
- Identify what is particularly important for and to the young person and prioritise accordingly.
- Support the young person's anxiety (and your own).
- Work together and negotiate.
- Manage demands.
- Adapt.
- Allow the child/young person control in areas of their life where this is reasonable.

A priority is supporting the other people in the young person's environment to understand their needs and accept reasonable adjustments.

---

It is helpful to remember that the young person:

Can't, not won't.

---

 **Useful resources**

The PDA Society has helpful support: www.pdasociety.org.uk, including "Helpful approaches..." downloads for parents and teaching professionals

*Autism, Girls, & Keeping It All Inside* (Autistic Girls Network, 2022)

Initial Clinical Guidelines for Co-Occurring Autism Spectrum Disorder and Gender Dysphoria or Incongruence in Adolescents (Strang et al., 2018)

*Right from the Start: A Guide to Autism in the Early Years* (Ambitious About Autism, 2020)

The Coventry Grid version 2 (2015) is available online

## Severity

Parents are often keen to know the severity of their child's autism. Support needs are documented as part of the diagnosis if the DSM-5 criteria are used. It is challenging to make it meaningful. Not only does the profile change for children and young people over time, but individuals can also be more or less challenged in different situations. The impact on the environment is critical. Severity is a problematic concept: it may be relatively straightforward to identify severity in a young person with autism and severe learning difficulties who needs a high level of support across the day.

In school: George is expected to sit with peers in a busy classroom, the acoustics are not ideal and the lighting and ventilation (smells) are not in his direct control. The teacher directs tasks. These are differentiated to his interests with the aim to make them explicitly relevant to his life. He can participate in differentiated activities with some adjustments. His anxiety is moderate/high (distracted by sensory needs, language processing and social demands). His support needs appear moderate as he participates, but he could achieve more if he were less anxious: he tends to shut down and withdraw into his thoughts about gaming when overwhelmed.

In school:

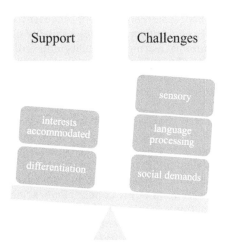

At home: George likes to spend time on his laptop constructing "mods" on interactive games. He is highly skilled, focused, independent and able to interact with peers through messaging (asynchronous preference). Sensory demands are low (preferred clothing, background noise and lighting controlled, comfortable seating, he has used a clean toilet with no driers, so he is happy to have a drink and is no longer thirsty). His anxiety is low, and his support needs are very low.

## Summary

- Diagnosis **must** be part of a multidisciplinary team. A speech and language therapist will be a part of that team.
- Identifying the strengths and needs of a child/young person is a critical part of the assessment.

## References

Abrahamson, V. et al., 2020. Realist Evaluation of Autism ServiCe Delivery (RE-ASCeD): Which Diagnostic Pathways Work Best, for Whom and in What Context? Protocol for a Rapid Realist Review. *BMJ Open*, 10(7). doi: http://dx.doi.org/10.1136/bmjopen-2020-037846

Abrahamson, V. et al., 2021. Realist Evaluation of Autism ServiCe Delivery (RE-ASCeD): Which Diagnostic Pathways Work Best, for Whom and in What Context? Findings from a Rapid Realist Review. *BMJ Open*, 11(e051241). doi: http://dx.doi.org/10.1136/bmjopen-2021-051241

Ambitious About Autism, 2020. *Right from the Start: A Guide to Autism in the Early Years*. [Online] Available at: https://www.ambitiousaboutautism.org.uk/information-about-autism/early-years/parent-toolkit [Accessed 02 10 2020].

American Psychiatric Association, 2000. *Diagnostic and Statistical Manual of Mental Disorders: DSM-IV*. Washington: American Psychiatric Association.

American Psychiatric Association, 2013. *Diagnostic and Statistical Manual of Mental Disorders*. Fifth ed. Washington: American Psychiatric Association.

Autistic Girls Network, 2022. *Autism, Girls, & Keeping It All Inside*. [Online] Available at: https://autisticgirlsnetwork.org/wp-content/uploads/2022/03/Keeping-it-all-inside.pdf [Accessed 22 7 2022].

Autistica, n.d. a *Anxiety and Autism*. [Online] Available at: https://www.autistica.org.uk/what-is-autism/signs-and-symptoms/anxiety-and-autism [Accessed 06 03 2021].

Autistica, n.d. b *Depression and Autism*. [Online] Available at: https://www.autistica.org.uk/what-is-autism/signs-and-symptoms/depression-and-autism [Accessed 05 03 2021].

Autistica, n.d. c *Learning Disability and Autism*. [Online] Available at: https://www.autistica.org.uk/what-is-autism/signs-and-symptoms/learning-disability-and-autism [Accessed 23 10 2022].

Bishop, D. V. et al., 2017. Phase 2 of CATALISE: A multinational and multidisciplinary Delphi consensus study of problems with language development: Terminology. *The Journal of Child Psychology and Psychiatry*, 58(10), p. 1068–1080.

Bryan, K., Freer, J. & Furlong, C., 2007. Language and Communication Difficulties in Juvenile Offenders. *International Journal of Language and Communication Disorders*, 42(5), pp. 505–520.

Criminal Justice Joint Inspection, 2021. *Neurodiversity in the Criminal Justice System: A Review of Evidence*. [Online] Available at: https://www.justiceinspectorates.gov.uk/hmicfrs/publications/neurodiversity-in-the-criminal-justice-system/ [Accessed 18 08 2022].

ECC (Embracing Complexity Coalition), 2019a. *Embracing Complexity in Diagnosis: Multi-Diagnostic Pathways for Neurodevelopmental Conditions*. London: Embracing Complexity Coalition.

ECC (Embracing Complexity Coalition), 2019b. *Embracing Complexity: Towards New Approaches for Supporting People with Neurodevelopmental Conditions*. [Online] Available at: https://embracingcomplexity.org.uk/assets/documents/Autistica-Embracing-Complexity-Report-Final.pdf [Accessed 29 03 2020].

Kallitsounaki, A. & Williams, D. M., 2022. Autism Spectrum Disorder and Gender Dysphoria/Incongruence. A Systematic Literature Review and Meta-Analysis. *Journal of Autism and Developmental Disorders*. doi: 10.1007/s10803-022-05517-y

Kindgren, E. Perez, A. Q., & Knez, R., 2021. Prevalence of ADHD and Autism Spectrum Disorder in Children with Hypermobility Spectrum Disorders or Hypermobile Ehlers–Danlos Syndrome: A Retrospective Study. *Neuropsychiatric Disease and Treatment*, 17, p. 379–388.

Lord, C., 2014. *Interactive Autism Network: Frequently Asked Questions about Autism Spectrum Diagnosis*. [Online] Available at: https://iancommunity.org/cs/articles/frequently_asked_questions_about_autism_spectrum_diagnoses [Accessed 05 10 2020].

Lord, C. et al., 2012. *Autism Diagnostic Observation Schedule*, 2nd edition. London: Pearson.

Milton, D., 2013. *'Natures Answer to Over-Conformity': Deconstructing Pathological Demand Avoidance.* [Online] Available at: https://kar.kent.ac.uk/62694/ [Accessed 19 09 2022].

Moran, H., 2010. Clinical Observations of the Differences between Children on the Autism Spectrum and Those with Attachment Problems: The Coventry Grid. *Good Autism Practice,* 11(2), pp. 44–57.

National Institute for Health and Care Excellence, 2020. *Autism in Children: What Else Might It Be?* [Online] Available at: https://cks.nice.org.uk/topics/autism-in-children/diagnosis/differential-diagnosis/ [Accessed 21 02 2021].

National Institute of Health and Care Excellence (NICE), 2017. *Autism Spectrum Disorder in under 19s: Recognition, Referral and Diagnosis. Clinical Guideline [CG128].* [Online] Available at: https://www.nice.org.uk/guidance/cg128 [Accessed 08 08 2020].

NHS England, 2019. *The NHS Long Term Plan.* Redditch: NHS England.

Roman-Urrestarazu, A. et al., 2021. Association of Race/Ethnicity and Social Disadvantage with Autism Prevalence in 7 Million School Children in England. *JAMAPediatrics,* 29(3), p. e210054.

Rong, Y., Yang, C.-J., Jin, Y. & Wang, Y., 2021. Prevalence of Attention-deficit/Hyperactivity Disorder in Individuals with Autism Spectrum Disorder: A Meta-analysis. *Research in Autism Spectrum Disorders,* 83.

Royal College of Speech and Language Therapists, n.d. *Autism – Guidance.* [Online] Available at: https://www.rcslt.org/members/clinical-guidance/autism/autism-guidance/ [Accessed 18 02 2021].

Rutter, M., LeCouteur, A. & Lord, C., 2003. *Autism Diagnostic Interview, Revised.* London: Pearson.

Santorer, L. A. et al., 2020. Felt but not seen: Observed restricted repetitive behaviors are associated with self-report-but not parent-report-obsessive-compulsive disorder symptoms in youth with autism spectrum disorder. *Autism,* 24(4), pp. 983–994.

Steffenburg, H., Steffenburg, S., Gillberg, C. & Billstedt, E., 2018. Children with Autism Spectrum Disorders and Selective Mutism. *Neuropsychiatric Disease and Treatment,* 14, pp. 1163–1169.

Strang, J. F. et al., 2018. Initial Clinical Guidelines for Co-Occurring Autism Spectrum Disorder and Gender Dysphoria or Incongruence in Adolescents. *Journal of Clinical Child & Adolescent Psychology,* 47(1), pp. 105–115.

Wikramanayake, W. N. M. et al., 2018. Autism Spectrum Disorders in Adult Outpatients with Obsessive Compulsive Disorder in the UK. *International Journal of Psychiatry in Clinical Practice,* 22(1), pp. 54–62.

Williams, M. E., Fink, C. & Zamor, I., 2013. Autism Assessment in Children with Optic Nerve Hypoplasia and Other Visual Impairments. *Developmental Medicine and Child Neurology* 56(1), pp. 66–72

World Health Organisation, 2021. *ICD-11 Autism Spectrum Disorder.* [Online] Available at: https://icd.who.int/browse11/l-m/en#/http%3a%2f%2fid.who.int%2ficd%2fentity%2f437815624 [Accessed 17 06 2021].

World Health Organization, 2022. *International Classification of Diseases Eleventh Revision (ICD-11).* 11th ed. Geneva: World Health Organization.

Young, S. et al., 2020. Guidance for Identification and Treatment of Individuals with Attention Deficit/Hyperactivity Disorder and Autism Spectrum Disorder based upon Expert Consensus. *BMC Medicine,* 18(146), p. 146.

Zampella, C. J. et al., 2021. Motor Skill Differences in Autism Spectrum Disorder: A Clinically Focused Review. *Current Psychiatry Reports,* 23(64), 64.

# SECTION II
# What to do

# IDENTIFICATION OF NEEDS

DOI: 10.4324/9781003154334-5

**Key points**

Identifying needs allows the opportunity to remove barriers and provide relevant support.

**Focus on identification of needs**

- Autonomy/self-advocacy:
  - Is support needed for the individual to express preferences and opinions and to make choices?
  - What are the individual's priorities?
- Understanding autism:
  - Who needs support?
    - Child/young person.
    - Family.
    - Education setting (school/early years/other).
    - Community.
- Needs that may be associated with autism:
  - Communication: means, reasons, opportunities.
  - Distressed behaviour.
  - Emotional regulation.
  - Perspective-taking.
  - Sensory needs.

# Introduction

Prioritising needs is challenging when working with autistic children and young people. It depends on a combination of individual factors, including what the family, school and community understand about autism generally and the priorities and needs of the individual and the people around them. Often, the empathy of the key people in the individual's life and their autonomy in implementing support significantly impact positive outcomes.

| Differences ≠ needs |
| --- |

All autistic children and young people will have differences in communication, sensory processing and information processing. Identifying their needs should be an outcome of their diagnostic assessment, but the focus is not to work towards the youngster behaving like a neurotypical person. The impact of these needs can be significant, affecting wellbeing and participation. For example:

- A task might be easy one day but impossible another.
- A young person might be independent in some aspects of life but have unexpected gaps (e.g. continence), often referred to as a "spiky profile."
- Particular interests may lead other people to overestimate an individual's ability in other areas (e.g. in-depth knowledge about history but unable to engage in play with a peer).
- The team may have different priorities.

## Early intervention

Early intervention is widely discussed as an aspiration for children with a new diagnosis of autism or likely to have autism. This premise continues throughout life. It is not just early in the child or the young person's life but early in the issues that arise. For example, the transition to secondary education at age 11 for most pupils in the United Kingdom is a crucial time. Early planning for the young person, school and family will make a difference in the child's adaptation to the new school.

Particular times to actively review needs include:

- Starting school.
- Secondary transfer.
- Puberty.
- Move into adulthood:
  - Child → adult health/care services.
  - Education → work.
  - School → college.
- Life events:
  - Separation: end of own close relationships or those close to the individual.
  - Significant illness of loved ones.
  - New diagnoses (e.g. autism).
  - Death of loved ones (including pets).
  - Marriage of loved ones.
  - New birth (e.g. new siblings).
  - New school.
  - Moving house, etc.

Consider the child/young person's strengths and support needs at these times proactively. Focus on their interests and consider further developing support that has previously been effective. The National Autistic Society (www.autism.org.uk) has support and advice on many issues. See section titled "Social understanding" in Chapter 5.

## Essential for family and carers: understand autism

Following a diagnosis, support for the parent/carer to understand autism and what this means for their child can be part of the role of the speech and language therapist (SLT). This may be part of a formal post-diagnosis offer (e.g. the National Autistic Society EarlyBird, EarlyBird Plus or Teen Life programmes or a local offer).

## What to do

Identify the support needed for the young person to understand their autism to support their autonomy and self-advocacy.

Observation of the child/young person in a familiar environment and discussion with people who know the young person provide important information about their needs. Many profiles exist that autism teams can use effectively, e.g. evidence based and highly regarded SCERTS® (Prizant et al., 2006), including the freely available online AET Progression Framework (Autism Education Trust, 2019). It is always important to keep in mind that the focus is on strengths and needs and not identifying differences.

---

Understanding and using the child's strengths and having a profile of their needs allow for personalised support.

---

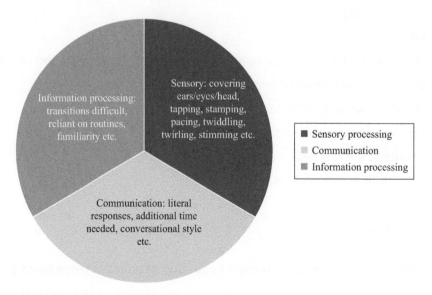

**FIGURE 3.1** Autism: relative needs, equal.

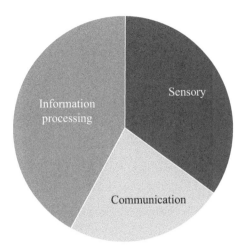

**FIGURE 3.2** Relative needs, unequal: communication needs are less, but the impact of information processing and sensory needs is likely to mean that the young person does find communication extremely challenging until other needs are supported.

Estimating the relative impact of sensory, communication and information processing needs helps identify strategies. If a young person is overwhelmed by their sensory environment, they will be unable to process other information effectively. Collaboration with other professionals to identify needs and plan support is crucial.

## Communication: means, reasons and opportunities

Money and Thurman's communication means, reasons and opportunities (Money & Thurman, 2002) model is helpful to support understanding communication needs and to communicate these to people working with the child/young person, whether or not the youngster has additional language needs.

### Means

For communication to be successful, a young person needs an effective **means** of expressing themselves:

The *Communication Matrix* (Rowland, 2022) provides an evidence-based framework for identifying the strengths and needs of children and young people at an early stage of communication or using forms of communication other than speaking or writing (communicationmatrix.org).

Needs in other aspects of language and communication should be identified:

Observation, ideally in several familiar settings (structured and unstructured).

> **Opportunities:** The young person needs an environment that facilitates communication: any resource or equipment needed is available, and people are responsive. Everyone in the young person's environment has a responsibility to support communication: by how they communicate and by embedding the use of strategies, teaching skills and removing barriers.

> **Means:** The young person needs a method of communication which may be any or all of speech, symbols, body language, gestures, signing, writing etc.

> **Reasons:** The young person needs a purpose for communication: to greet, ask for information, express feelings etc.

FIGURE 3.3 Communication: means, reasons and opportunities. (Money & Thurman, 2002)

Carer reports and assessments are valid for assessing expressive and receptive language skills in autistic children (Nordahl-Hansen et al., 2014).

Assessment tools suggested for assessing needs for diagnosis are useful (Chapter 2, pp. 38–39).

Superficially good expressive language can mask difficulties with understanding spoken language. Non-literal or context-dependent language may be particularly challenging. Speech and language delay or disorder can co-occur with autism, and any associated needs should be identified.

**What support is needed to develop means to communicate across the week?**

---------------------------------------------------------------------------------------------------------

## Reasons

Whatever a youngster's method of communication, they need to have autonomy: be able to communicate for a range of reasons, both functional and social.

Generally, schools focus greatly on listening, following instructions, requesting, commenting and reporting/retelling. We need to ensure that opportunities for other reasons are available. See Figure 3.4 and Table 3.1 for examples.

**What support is needed to develop reasons to communicate across the week?**

---------------------------------------------------------------------------------------------------------

## Opportunities

Looking at the child/young person's environment is critical to an assessment. What is it that helps/hinders the youngster's communication? Finding out about their communication

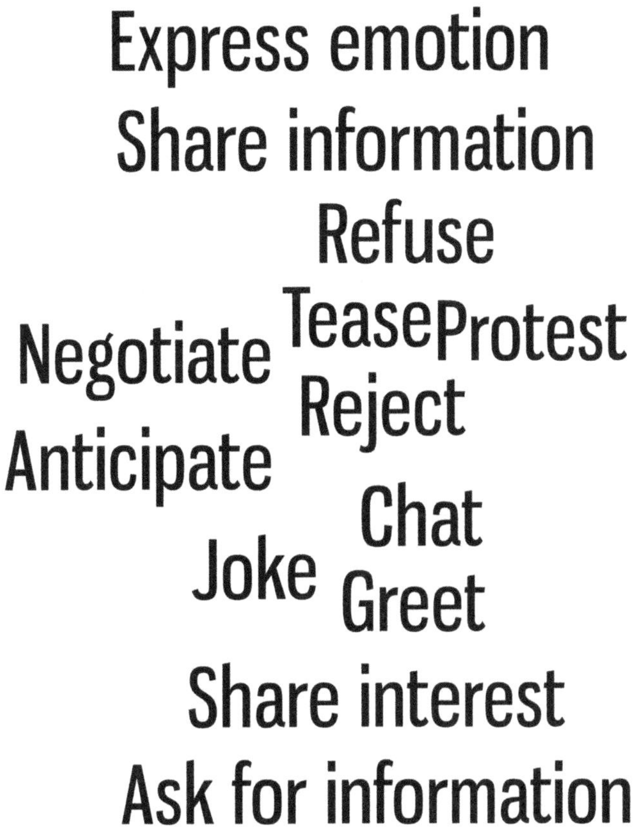

# Express emotion
# Share information
# Refuse
# Negotiate Tease Protest
# Reject
# Anticipate
# Chat
# Joke Greet
# Share interest
# Ask for information

**FIGURE 3.4** Word cloud: communication reasons.

in different settings and with different people provides valuable information about their needs.

**What support is needed to develop communication opportunities/remove barriers across the week?**

## Voice of the child

Children and young people with autism vary in their ability to express their thoughts and opinions. A fundamental part of the SLT's role includes supporting the young person to be able to express themselves, and this is a focus throughout. Supporting a child or young person to be able to express themselves can be complex and depends upon the youngster.

## Talking Mats

Talking Mats is a research-based communication tool that helps people to organise their thoughts and express their views (Talking Mats, 2022). It is beneficial for many children and young people to give their opinion without relying on expressive language and

**TABLE 3.1** Communication: reasons and means

| Means ↓ / Reasons → | | Notes (e.g. examples, coordination of strategies) | Request: Object | Activity | Help | More | Attention | Affection | Reassurance | Information | Refuse/reject |
|---|---|---|---|---|---|---|---|---|---|---|---|
| Symbolic | Speech | | | | | | | | | | |
| | Sign | | | | | | | | | | |
| | Symbol | | | | | | | | | | |
| | Object | | | | | | | | | | |
| Conventional | Vocalisation | | | | | | | | | | |
| | Eye gaze | | | | | | | | | | |
| | Facial expression | | | | | | | | | | |
| | Nod/shake head | | | | | | | | | | |
| | Point (contact/distant) | | | | | | | | | | |
| | Wave | | | | | | | | | | |
| Intentional | Take hand | | | | | | | | | | |
| | Give | | | | | | | | | | |
| | Push | | | | | | | | | | |
| | Reach | | | | | | | | | | |
| | Touch (hug) | | | | | | | | | | |
| Pre-intentional | Proximity | | | | | | | | | | |
| | Crying/screaming | | | | | | | | | | |
| | Escape | | | | | | | | | | |
| | Self-injury/hurting | | | | | | | | | | |
| | Not observed | | | | | | | | | | |

| | Notes | Comment | Share information | Social routine (greet, please) | Direct attention | Protest | Negotiate | Tease/joke | Report/retell | Share interest | Express/share emotions | Anticipate | Social/chat/other |
|---|---|---|---|---|---|---|---|---|---|---|---|---|---|
| Speech | | | | | | | | | | | | | |
| Sign | | | | | | | | | | | | | |
| Symbol | | | | | | | | | | | | | |
| Object | | | | | | | | | | | | | |
| Vocal. | | | | | | | | | | | | | |
| Eye ga. | | | | | | | | | | | | | |
| F. exp. | | | | | | | | | | | | | |
| Nod/sh. | | | | | | | | | | | | | |
| Point | | | | | | | | | | | | | |
| Wave | | | | | | | | | | | | | |
| T. ha. | | | | | | | | | | | | | |
| Give | | | | | | | | | | | | | |
| Push | | | | | | | | | | | | | |
| Reach | | | | | | | | | | | | | |
| Touch | | | | | | | | | | | | | |
| Prox. | | | | | | | | | | | | | |
| Cry/scr. | | | | | | | | | | | | | |
| Escape | | | | | | | | | | | | | |
| Self-inj. | | | | | | | | | | | | | |
| Not ob. | | | | | | | | | | | | | |

Key: Ⓢ spontaneous, Ⓟ prompted, Ⓘ imitated.

conversation. This can include how the individual feels about different situations, for example, expressing an opinion (e.g. like/don't like, worried/not worried, I can do it/I need help) in different situations (e.g. free time/school/transition to secondary school/independence skills). Having completed a Talking Mat, the person supporting the individual checks that they have understood, giving the individual the opportunity to reflect and change their mind and then highlight areas they would like to change.

The Talking Mats social enterprise sells digital and physical resources and training to support staff in using Talking Mats to help people with communication difficulties express themselves in health, education, social care and residential settings: www.talkingmats.com.

For young people who cannot complete a Talking Mat (approximately Blank level 2 or two keyword understanding required), views can be sought by observing their preferences

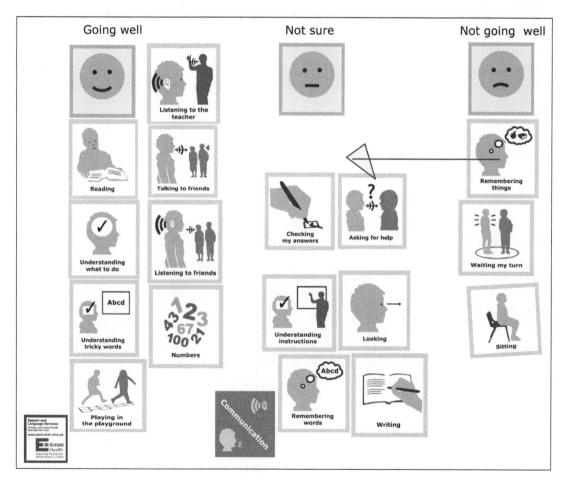

**FIGURE 3.5** Talking Mat: communication strengths and needs.

This young person identified that they would like to improve their ability to remember things, so strategies were agreed upon and a target set.

alongside seeking information from parents and carers. This can be documented with annotated photos of preferences.

Some youngsters may have developed strategies to help manage situations or activities they find challenging (e.g. stimming). These strategies are not preferred activities but regulation strategies. Unpicking these can be tricky.

---

**VOICE OF CHILD**

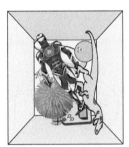

I enjoy exploring the classroom:

I found the choosing box and enjoyed briefly playing with the sensory ball, popper (jumping) toy, dinosaur and microphone. I explored these by looking, holding and tapping.

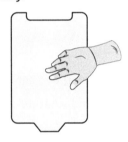

I knew where to find a box of soft toys. I held SpongeBob for a few seconds, explored him, and emptied the box.

I enjoyed tapping the bottom and sides of the box and listening to / feeling the effects. I looked and smiled when an adult joined in tapping with me.

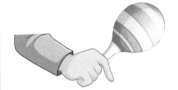

I enjoyed the musical instrument box: pressing buttons to make tunes play, shaking and tapping.

I enjoyed holding, watching and tapping the sand timer. I was interested for 5 minutes. Later, with help, I was able to move on from watching the sand timer to go outside.

 I use my ear defenders when I'm anxious, in busy places or when the noise level rises. I didn't use them while exploring these resources.

---

Parents and carers are important in expressing their thoughts about the child's priorities, although caution is required around understanding what is <u>important to</u> their child (e.g. watching Minecraft on YouTube) rather than what they feel is <u>important for</u> them (having a conversation with a friend).

## Self-advocacy

Self-advocacy is the ability to express one's own needs and the actions needed to meet these needs. For effective self-advocacy, the young person must have insight into their own strengths and needs.

Steps:

- **Modelling**: ensure that people are talking about things that are difficult for them (*not the autistic child*) and what helps ("I can't draw straight lines, I'll use a ruler," "I can't remember all that, I'll take a photo," "I can't hear while Fred's talking, let's go shut the door," "I'm <u>tired</u>, I need <u>water</u>").

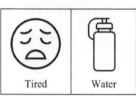

- **Noticing** and **reflecting**: things that the youngster is good at, what they find challenging and what helps.

  Developing this into a communication passport (CALL Scotland, 2022) ensures that the information is accessible.

> A communication passport is a highly personalised document that belongs to the individual. It includes important information about them that they can share with other people. This will include a positive introduction, including strengths, interests and their communication style, what they need from their communication partner and their support needs.

- **Teaching skills and providing scripts** can be helpful: "no, I don't like...," "I don't want...," "stop," "I need...," "it helps when...."
- **Prompting**: asking, "What do you need?"

Self-advocacy accompanied by an autistic communication style may be perceived as inappropriate. This is a double empathy issue (see p. 71), and the blame for communication breakdown must not be placed on the autistic young person. Ensuring that both parties understand the reason for the communication breakdown will support mutual understanding and allow an exploration of alternative strategies for both sides.

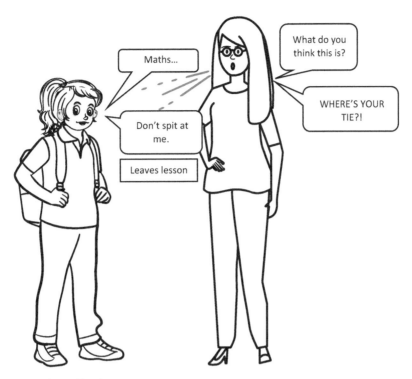

**FIGURE 3.6** Rachel's self-advocacy.

**TABLE 3.2** Rachel's self-advocacy

| Teacher's perspective | Rachel's perspective |
|---|---|
| • Another pupil broke the uniform code. <br> • Insolent (answering back). <br> • Public false accusation (spitting) to undermine me. <br> • Left lesson (more disrespect). | • I just answered the question (literal understanding). Didn't infer the hidden question about her school uniform. Has permission to remove tie, reasonable adjustment for sensory differences. <br> • Teacher was standing too close, saliva on my clothes; I asked her to stop. <br> • Teacher was speaking too loud, causing sensory overload. |
| With a better understanding of neurodivergent needs: | |
| Providing more personal space and a quieter voice: "Rachel, where's your tie?" | "In my bag." Rachel passes her teacher a permission slip excusing her from the uniform rule due to sensory differences associated with autism (a "reasonable adjustment"). |

## Summary

As autistic children and young people are a heterogeneous group, it is difficult to iden-tify clear-cut evidence-based practice. It is increasingly agreed that relying on the "gold standard" of randomised controlled trials does not always provide the best information about support for an individual (Best et al., 2019). The choice of intervention should be informed by the identification of needs. Ensuring that the child/young person's voice is central to identifying needs is critical.

## Useful resources

*2019 Progression Framework* (Autism Education Trust, 2019)

*All About Me: A Step-by-Step Guide to Telling Children and Young People on the Autism Spectrum about Their Diagnosis* (Miller, 2018)

*Autism, Identity and Me: A Practical Workbook and Professional Guide to Empower Autistic Children and Young People* (Duffus, 2023)

*Communication Matrix* (Rowland, 2022)

*Communication Passports* (www.communicationpassports.org.uk)

*The SCERTS® Manual: A Comprehensive Educational Approach for Children with Autism Spectrum Disorders* (Prizant et al., 2006)

## References

Autism Education Trust, 2019. *2019 Progression Framework*. [Online] Available at: https://www.autismeducationtrust.org.uk/resources/progression-framework [Accessed 14 10 2020].

Best, W., Ping Sze, W., Edmundson, A. & Nickels, L., 2019. What Counts as Evidence? Swimming against the Tide: Valuing both Clinically Informed Experimentally Controlled Case Series and Randomized Controlled Trials in Intervention Research. *Evidence-Based Communication Assessment and Intervention*, 13(3), pp. 107-135.

Blank, M., Rose, S. A. & Berlin, L. J., 1978. *The Language of Learning: The Preschool Years*. Australia: Grune & Stratton.

CALL Scotland, 2022. *Personal Communication Passports*. [Online] Available at: https://www.communicationpassports.org.uk/Home/ [Accessed 10 10 2022].

Cullen, R., 2021. *The Autistic Communication Hypothesis*. [Online] Available at: https://aucademy.co.uk/rachel-cullen-they-them/ [Accessed 15 08 2022].

Duffus, R., 2023. *Autism, Identity and Me: A Practical Workbook and Professional Guide to Empower Autistic Children and Young People Aged 10+*. Abingdon: Routledge.

Miller, A., 2018. *All About Me: A Step-by-Step Guide to Telling Children and Young People on the Autism Spectrum about Their Diagnosis*. London: Jessica Kingley Publishers.

Money, D. & Thurman, S., 2002. Inclusive Communication – Coming Soon Near You? *Speech and language Therapy in Practice*, Autumn 2002, 4-6.

Nordahl-Hansen, A., Kaale, A. & Ulvund, S. E., 2014. Language Assessment in Children with Autism Spectrum Disorder: Concurrent Validity Between Report-based Assessments and Direct Tests. *Research in Autism Spectrum Disorders*, 8(9), pp. 1100-1106.

Prizant, B. M. et al., 2006. *The SCERTS® Model: A Comprehensive Educational Approach for Children with Autism Spectrum Disorders: Volume 1 Assessment*. Baltimore: Brookes.

Rowland, C., 2022. *Communication Matrix*. [Online] Available at: https://communicationmatrix.org/ [Accessed 14 10 2022].

Talking Mats, 2022. *Talking Mats: Improving Communication Improving Lives*. [Online] Available at: https://www.talkingmats.com/ [Accessed 24 10 2022].

Wiig, E. H., Semel, E. & Secord, W. A., 2013. *The Clinical Evaluation of Language Fundamentals - Fifth Edition (CELF-5 UK)*. Fifth ed. London: Pearson.

# SUPPORTING AUTISTIC CHILDREN AND YOUNG PEOPLE IN SCHOOL AND SOCIETY

DOI: 10.4324/9781003154334-6

**Key points**

The focus of this chapter is on the young person's environment.

- Staff to understand the impact of autism.
- Make the environment make sense.
  - Use people support – how individual people adapt to provide support.
  - Use environmental supports – how environments are supportive.
    - Consider sensory aspects.

**Focus on**

- Building positive relationships.
- Using visual supports, including objects, photos, pictures and symbols for various purposes.
- Developing social understanding: make unspoken social rules explicit. Develop mutual understanding. Support learning of skills, e.g. group-work skills (including oracy in school).
- Increasing communication opportunities.

## Introduction

"Many of us experience and interact with the world in different ways from others thanks to the make-up and behaviour of our brains" (Spiers, 2019). Where autism is seen as a difference rather than a disorder, with a different way of thinking and experiencing the world, a focus on understanding the individuals' specific learning style, needs, interests and preferences is vital. The speech and language therapist (SLT) has a role in identifying needs and supporting the child/young person in effectively sharing this information.

The National Strategy for Autistic Children, Young People and Adults 2021–2026 highlights that understanding and adapting to individuals' needs is the responsibility of all community members. The specific themes of the strategy are "improving understanding and acceptance of autism within society" and "improving autistic children and young people's access to education" (HM Government, 2021).

This chapter explores general principles and specific strategies to support autistic children in education before focusing on individualised needs in later chapters.

## Role of SLTs

The SLT may work with an autistic child/young person (see later chapters) but will also have a role in supporting those in the child's environment:

1.  Support the parents/carers/staff to develop relationships - see Chapters 5-8.
2.  Support parents/carers/staff to develop the environment to be communication/ autism-friendly.

## Double empathy problem

Many of the children and young people are known to SLTs have additional language (and learning) needs. Whether or not the youngster has additional needs, it is vital to take into account the impact of the double empathy problem (Milton, 2012). Both partners in an interaction between an autistic and neurotypical pair have challenges, and empathy is required on both sides.

NEED:

*   To develop a mutual understanding of cultures. Some autistic children and young people have learned a lot about the neurotypical culture as they live it; the neurotypical people in their lives probably have lots of catching up to do.
*   To develop an awareness of neurotypical vs autistic use of language.
*   To develop an awareness of the reason for problems (e.g. higher processing load, ambiguous language, social ambiguity) and avoid blaming the autistic youngster.

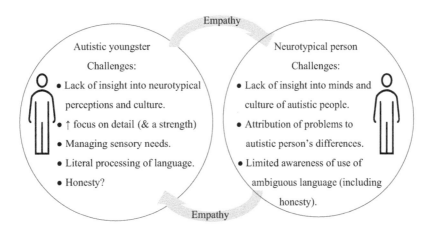

**FIGURE 4.1** Double empathy problem.

Individuals and settings can be encouraged to access training and to review their good practice using resources available online, for example:

- The Autism Education Trust Competency Framework for individual staff working with early years, school-aged and young people in post-16 education (Autism Education Trust, 2022).
- The Autism Education Trust Standards Framework supports the implementation of "Good Autism Practice" in early years settings, schools and post-16 settings (Autism Education Trust, 2022) or participation in ELKLAN's Communication Friendly Settings programme (ELKLAN, 2022).

Within the school setting, a whole-school focus on understanding autism has a critical impact on support. Both children and young people with and without additional speech, language and/or learning needs need support.

Some support elements are likely to benefit most autistic children and young people (and many others).

- Staff to understand autism generally, with the opportunity to personalise this learning to individuals.
- Staff to understand the child and their autism: clear descriptions of strengths, preferences and needs available to staff to support positive relationships. Ensure communication passport/pen portrait/pupil profile is available and up to date.

Resources are now available to support primary schools to teach pupils about neurodiversity so that pupils can learn about brain-based differences in how we learn, think and experience the world (Alcorn et al., 2022).

## In school

Schools in England and beyond must make their environment and learning opportunities accessible. **Ordinarily available provision** includes quality teaching and interaction, which supports children from the school's usual resources. **Additional and different** provision is made when a youngster needs extra support that is more specialised and may require more physical adaptations and/or specialist intervention (e.g. speech and language therapy, occupational therapy, autism advisory team).

The *Code of Practice* (Department for Education and Department of Health, 2015) links high-quality teaching with ordinarily available provision, explaining that "higher quality teaching ordinarily available to the whole class" will mean that few children will need specialist intervention.

The Equality Act (2010) does not permit discrimination based on disability. However, it allows for more favourable treatment of disabled people to avoid them being at a substantial disadvantage (known as "reasonable adjustment").

Teaching and mediating learning is the responsibility of the school. Various documents support school staff in knowing their responsibilities and with general strategies for children and young people with a range of needs, including autism; for example, the London Borough of Enfield's "Ordinarily Available Provision" (Enfield Council, 2022).

SLTs can support as part of the graduated approach used in schools (assess, plan, do, review).

Universal/wave 1: Quality First Teaching through universal strategies, e.g. training: identifying pupils with additional needs; developing and supporting the development of whole-school strategies/support.

Targeted/wave 2: supporting the school to implement targeted interventions, which might be the school delivering small-group interventions.

Specialist/wave 3: supporting a specific programme for a pupil, delivered by a member of the school staff (supervised by the SLT) or the SLT.

This section focuses on teaching and interaction from the school's usual resources (ordinarily available provision).

Communication Friendly Settings (ELKLAN, www.elklan.co.uk) provide school staff with knowledge and skills to teach pupils with speech, language and communication needs, including autism. The teacher is responsible for differentiation, ensuring that all pupils have understood. This will include supporting learning so that it is broken down as needed and activities are designed to maintain the interest and attention of all pupils.

### ENGAGEMENT IS KEY TO PARTICIPATION AND LEARNING

Relationships: a focus on relationships supports engagement, for example, as part of the personal, social, health and citizenship education (PSHCE) curriculum. Some autistic pupils have prosopagnosia, so they do not recognise people by their faces. Photo IDs and displays with photos and names are helpful to support where this is tricky.

Interests: use irresistible activities to engage the young person (see Chapter 5).

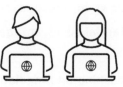

The young person's interests can be extremely helpful in engaging them.

Children and young people with autism need the people around them to have high expectations of their understanding and competence; however, alongside this, support must be available as needed.

## Visual support

Many children and young people are helped by visual support. Visual information stays and is consistent, whereas auditory information is transitory. It is usually helpful to support auditory information with visual information, which is likely to aid processing and allow checking back. However a person tries to consistently repeat information verbally, they may well change the wording a little. Even if this is not the case, the intonation, speed and volume may differ, so the young person may have to restart the processing as if the words are entirely new. If visual information is provided, then this will remain constant.

The purpose of visual supports is to help understanding.

## Visual supports are universal

Visual support helps in understanding spoken language. We might use different aspects to support understanding (and expression) at different times. For example, we might:

- Use photos at the barber to choose a hairstyle from a poster.
- Use pictures to help us understand the menu in an unfamiliar language (risky!).
- Show a cup to offer a drink in a noisy room if we expect that the offer might not be heard.
- Gesture to discretely remind someone of the expectations (finger to lips to remind a child to be quiet when grandma is talking).
- Look at objects and signs, so we know where to cross the road safely.

Visual supports can be confusing if symbols are ambiguous or overwhelming (e.g. the symbol does not share a resemblance with an item, the same symbol is used for different purposes or too many symbols are used).

---

"Symbol" is used as a broad term to describe any representation of something (e.g. an object or idea) by something else (e.g. a spoken, signed or written word, a photo, drawing or object).

"Symbol" is also used as a narrow term to describe symbols used in picture support, e.g.

---

Many people rely on support, often visual, to get through life. A busy life or anxiety can increase reliance on support. People develop strategies that are workable and helpful. For some people, this involves apps on a smartphone; for others, a note is jotted on their calendar. Developing helpful strategies can take experimentation and perseverance.

## Universal visual supports

- Lists (paper or virtual), for example:
  - Shopping lists.
  - To-do lists.
  - Celebration invitation.
  - Gifts planned/bought for people and received.
  - Planning lists (pilots, anaesthetists and other highly skilled professionals have regimented, mandatory checklists to ensure that safety is maintained).
- Mnemonics help many people. They may be well known (Naughty Elephants Squirt Water: sequence of compass directions, or rhymes: "30 days has September"). Highly personal mnemonics can be memorable ("Mr Verocan Eats Jam Sandwiches Under Neath Pianos" – planets of the solar system when Pluto was a planet!).

- Calendars or diaries: paper or virtual, which might include notifications and alarms.
- Alarm set: a reminder to get up, take medication, school run, attend an appointment or buy pizza toppings.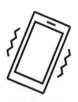
- Text reminder: send a scheduled message: cancel a subscription, make a phone call, make an appointment.
- Signposts.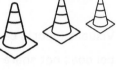
- Warning signs: e.g. slippery floor, danger, CCTV, guard dog.
- Locating items (putting packed lunch by the front door, Post-it notes on the door as a reminder).
- Objects: sink, soap and paper towels adjacent to the toilet, which might remind about handwashing.
- Own phone number taped onto laptop and phone.
- Writing a reminder on hand.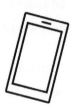
- Taking a photo on the phone (e.g. instructions, description, code and location).
- Maps/GPS directions/what3words.
- Voice note on the phone.
- Coloured towels, lunch boxes, etc., for different family members, groups, etc.
- YouTube instruction videos.
- Furniture assembly diagrams.
- Storage organisation (pants on the left, socks on the right), shelves/drawers labelled with word, image, outline, code (library).
- Patterns for pin codes, keyboard clues for passwords (@ for a, 5 for s or patterns).
- Signals from other people. For example, finger to lips: sh/zip lips = be quiet (don't talk about that!); mime wipe mouth (you've got some food on your lips); "XYZ" (eXamine Your Zip – zip it up!).

The 2020 coronavirus pandemic led to a considerable increase in signposting (e.g. where to stand, what to wear, how to interact). The clarity this provided around the expectations as the lockdown lifted benefited everybody.

Visual supports suggested for children and young people with autism may be similar to these, or they may be more specialised in nature. The idea is that they will support the youngster in understanding and may help develop independence.

Once a child's needs have been identified, visual supports can help. These often support communication needs but may also relate to other specific issues associated with autism. Some supports may be generic, while others may require much personalisation.

Visual supports can help an autistic youngster by

- Helping understand language and social ambiguity.
- Making life more predictable, providing structure and routines.
- Reducing reliance on prompting from other people.
- Supporting memory.
- Increasing confidence.
- Reducing anxiety and frustration.
- Supporting opportunities to interact with others.

## Ordinarily available visual support in the classroom

Visual supports are common in most classrooms, particularly in the early years and early primary education. As these children are at the early stages of reading, teachers use written words to label items to support reading and support written words with images for many purposes:

- Labelling: coat pegs/drawers.
- Organisation: outline of resources traced onto a shelf so that resources are tidied away properly.
- Routines: use visual supports to help young children understand the structure of the school day (e.g. visual timetable).
- Social understanding, the expectations in school (handwashing, listening to each other, hand up, etc.).
- Colour-coded visual support for language (e.g. colourful semantics) so that question words are colour coded to support understanding and organisation of spoken language.
- Word mats, timelines, flashcards, posters, mind maps and storyboards.

To understand these, all pupils may need some teaching. A timetable displayed on a wall may only influence pupils if it is introduced and actively used. Noticing and rewarding children using visual supports can be powerful. Focusing on what the children/young people should be doing is important (walk in the corridors rather than "no running"). This *ordinarily available* provision will help all children, including many of those with additional needs. However, autistic children and young people may need *more personalised support* to participate in all aspects of school life. Autistic children and young people, particularly those with additional language and/or learning needs, are likely to need these visual supports to be sustained throughout their education.

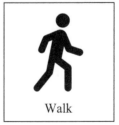
Walk

## More personalised visual support

Many children and young people, including those with autism, rely on prompting to participate. Supporting all children to increase their independence and participation remains appropriate. Strategies including visual support may be beneficial to avoid over-reliance on prompting from another person. This may need to be more specialised than the strategies typically used. For example, there may be a class timetable for all children in a primary classroom. Some pupils may need a personalised timetable that breaks the day down further and incorporates their interests. A small number of children may need an individualised timetable that dovetails with the class timetable to support their understanding and participation:

- Understanding the routines.
- Incorporating their interests to make the routines meaningful.
- Understanding the time concepts: how long are different expectations? Support to understand time by teaching with clocks and/or timers may be used.
- A five-minute break with access to their interest between learning activities to sustain motivation.

The type of support that helps depends on the individual.

Visual supports available to all can help with any speech, language and communication needs associated with autism (or other additional needs, e.g. social and emotional). These can include:

- **Sensory**: sensory needs are significant for many autistic children and young people. Careful identification of an individual's profile and accommodations to meet their needs is essential. The support of an occupational therapist is valuable in environmental assessment and essential in individual assessment and advice for youngsters with complex needs (see Chapter 7).
  - Prompts to proactively elicit discussion and accommodation of people's opinions and needs: modelling language and discussion of sensory preferences and needs: I like/don't like... sunny weather, this music, cold weather, the smell of soup cooking, wet trousers, thunder, etc.
  - Offers of available resources to support needs: ear defenders, shut the door, dry clothes, coat on, etc.
  - Prompts to share information: too noisy, too cold, hungry.
  - Prompts to request sensory support (break, weighted blanket, hand cream, ear defenders, movement break).

- **Communication:** including non-literal language.
  - Ambiguous words (sick, bad, dust, peer, bat) where context is needed to understand the meaning.
  - Prompts to request: I need ear defenders, turn the volume down, I need a break, water please.
  - Language board to go with a play activity.
  - Decision-making: use of decision-making tree.
  - Expressing preferences (as above).
  - Social understanding: highlighting the (social) context.
  - Perspective-taking: sharing own perspective with others and considering another person's point of view.
  - Organising information: categorising vocabulary, people's names and topic mats.
  - Social chit-chat.
  - Autonomy: expressing needs and problems (e.g. Figure 4.2 problem page).

- **Information processing**
  - A reminder of what is happening next (e.g. now – next [Figure 4.3], written schedule).
  - Transitions.
  - Routines: timetable, recurring events (e.g. handwashing, changing a library book).
  - Leisure/choices.
  - Expectations: supporting understanding of expectations e.g.
    - turn-taking (turn-taking wheel) so pupils (and teacher!) know when they are going to be asked a question, offered a turn etc

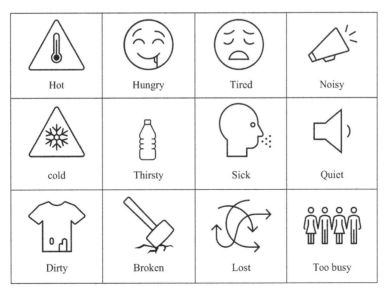

**FIGURE 4.2** Problem page.

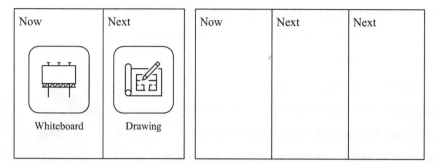

**FIGURE 4.3** Now – next.

- Learning group-working skills, including different roles (Lego® Therapy).
- Timekeeping (egg timer, clock with numbers and minute hand removed and picture of school/lunch/home added).

## The Engagement Model (Standards & Testing Agency, 2020)

This tool has become statutory for assessing primary-aged pupils in England working "below the standard of national curriculum assessments and not engaged in subject-specific study." It covers monitoring of progress in five areas:

- Exploration – exploring, including noticing and showing interest, e.g. by looking/reaching.
- Realisation – noticing that things happen and beginning to take some control to stop or change them.
- Anticipation – anticipating, including interpreting clues that an event will happen or finish: cause–effect.

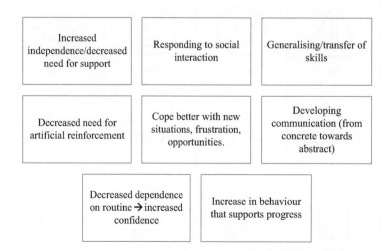

**FIGURE 4.4** Summary of types of progress that the Engagement Model might recognise.

- Persistence – sustaining attention.
- Initiation – starting an exploration/interaction.

Summarised from the Engagement Model (Standards & Testing Agency, 2020).

Monitoring these areas of progress can be relevant to any pupil and may provide additional information that may not be captured by the traditional review of targets.

## Community

We all live in a community. There are challenges for anyone in being part of a community. The challenges may seem overwhelming for autistic children and young people and their families. Relationship breakdown between parents of children with a disability is well known, adding to the complications of family life. Extended families are a vital source of support for many families, but supporting their understanding of differences and how to help could be useful.

Education settings, workplaces, clubs and leisure facilities are more aware of the need to support participation. Information is available on increasing accessibility in different settings. This has moved on from physical access, so there is increased awareness of and experience in meeting the needs of a diverse population. Parents often report that participation in the community is reliant on the empathy and flexibility of individuals and influential people in the community.

A communication-friendly environment involves:

- The physical setting.
- The people within the setting.

Families, playgroups, nurseries, schools and community groups all have a role to play in developing settings to make them welcoming for all. This might include clear explanations of the group's purpose, expectations and limitations and what support they can offer autistic participants and their families.

To consider the physical environment in detail is beyond the scope of this book. However, SLTs should be aware of the need to consider this and consult with an occupational therapist as needed. Consider the *Checklist for Autism Friendly Environments* (Simpson, 2016).

Within the United Kingdom, the Equality Act. (2010) expects public resources to make "reasonable adjustments" to be accessible to disabled people, including those with autism. Accessibility not only refers to physical adjustments but also to other means that make a setting inclusive.

Community facilities are more aware of the need to provide support for people with additional needs, including:

- Specific shopping times when lighting, noise levels and other sensory considerations are adapted to make the environment calmer.
- Provision for discrete ways that allow people to show that they might have additional support needs (like the sunflower lanyard).
- Visual: consideration of lighting (avoid fluorescent, be aware of reflected light, patterns of sunlight/shadow, moving blinds, sunlit dust in the environment), colours and patterns.
- Olfactory: consideration of smells of strongly scented items or cleaning products that can be seriously distracting.
- Auditory acoustics: an echo might be enjoyable, a distraction or an irritation, too much noise, distracting background noise (hum of projector, air circulation system, radiators) and noise signals (fire alarm, security system, sound effects on IT systems).
- Tactile: some young people have different preferences for fabrics, textures of food/ drinks and resources that can impact participation (e.g. stripping if made to wear non-preferred clothing).

## Planning and preparation

It can be challenging to control the environment when "out and about." Many families are helped by accessing "autism-friendly" opportunities (e.g. at leisure facilities: cinemas, trampoline parks, etc., some supermarkets have quieter sessions – fewer people and restricted noise on tannoys).

It can be helpful to prepare the child or young person in advance. Many places have resources to support this, and more generic support is available online. Local services may also be able to provide support (e.g. community dentist can be asked to provide a quieter, slower-paced appointment, or a child/young person can be referred to a special needs dentist).

Know the child:

- What do they need?
- How much information?

- In what format?
- Opportunity to read/discuss/rehearse/plan for changes? Use "now – next" (what we are doing now and then what is next) format.

---

**TOP TIPS FOR COMMUNICATION PARTNERS (PARENTS, CARERS, SCHOOL STAFF, ETC.)**

**Keep it short and simple** (KISS). Short sentences, simple vocabulary. Find out about the young person's understanding and use language at the level that the pupil understands (and teach/extend to the next level).

**Time to process.** Give the pupil plenty of time to process spoken language (count to ten slowly in your head before expecting a response).

**Model** an appropriate response (use peers).

**Say exactly what you mean.** Avoid ambiguous and/or non-literal language. Classroom management strategies may use humour (particularly in secondary schools). This may not be appropriate for pupils with language difficulties, including autism. It may cause extreme overt (e.g. answering back, anger, confusion) or covert (e.g. withdrawal, confusion, anxiety) responses.

**Use visual support** alongside spoken language. Show: use a demonstration, illustration or object.

**Use the pupil's interests** to encourage shared attention and participation.

**Respond to pupil**'s interaction/language. Repeat their word(s), protowords, "read" their symbols/signs and interpret their vocalisation as intentional communication.

REMEMBER the double empathy problem and strive to understand the other person's perspective.

---

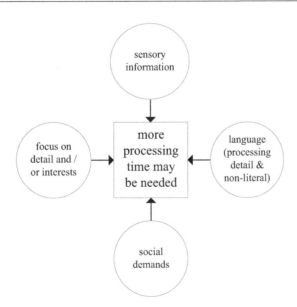

**FIGURE 4.5** Impact of differences on the processing time needed.

## Useful resources

*Autism and UK Airports – Improving Assistance for Passengers with Autism* (Fowler, 2022)

*Autism, Sport & Physical Activity* (Webster, 2016)

*Church for Everyone* (Rapley, 2022)

*My Health Passport* (National Autistic Society, 2017)

*Learning About Neurodiversity at School*: LEANS (Alcorn et al., 2022)
"A free programme for mainstream primary schools to introduce pupils aged 8–11 years to the concept of neurodiversity, and how it impacts our experiences at school"

*Checklist for Autism Friendly Environments*, endorsed by NICE and NAS (Simpson, 2016)

## References

Alcorn, A. M. et al., 2022. *Learning About Neurodiversity at School: A Resource Pack for Primary School Teachers and Pupils.* [Online] Available at: https://www.ed.ac.uk/salvesen-research/leans [Accessed 25 5 2022].

Autism Education Trust, 2022. *Framework Documents.* [Online] Available at: https://www.autismeducationtrust.org.uk/framework-documents [Accessed 12 10 2022].

Department for Education and Department of Health, 2015. *Special Educational Needs and Disability Code of Practice: 0 to 25 Years.* [Online] Available at: https://www.gov.uk/government/publications/send-code-of-practice-0-to-25 [Accessed 16 10 2022].

ELKLAN, 2022. *Communication Friendly Settings.* [Online] Available at: https://www.elklan.co.uk/OurWork/CaseStudies/CFSe/ [Accessed 15 10 2022].

Enfield Council, 2022. *Ordinarily Available Provision 2022–2025.* [Online] Available at: https://traded.enfield.gov.uk/news/2022/oct/ordinarily-available-provision-2022-2025 [Accessed 11 10 2022].

Equality Act 2010. [online] Available at: http://www.legislation.gov.uk/ukpga/2010/15/contents.

Fowler, A., 2022. *Autism and UK Airports – Improving Assistance for Passengers with Autism.* [Online] Available at: https://www.airport-parking-shop.co.uk/blog/uk-airports-need-step-assistance-autism/ [Accessed 25 10 2022].

HM Government, 2021. *The National Strategy for Autistic Children, Young People and Adults: 2021 to 2026.* London: HM Government.

Milton, D., 2012. On the Ontological Status of Autism: The 'Double Empathy Problem'. *Disability and Society,* 27(6), pp. 883–887.

National Autistic Society, 2017. *My Health Passport.* [Online] Available at: https://www.autism.org.uk/advice-and-guidance/topics/physical-health/my-health-passport [Accessed 25 10 2022].

Rapley, S., 2022. *Church for Everyone.* [Online] Available at: https://churchforeveryone.info/faith-autism/ [Accessed 25 10 2022].

Simpson, S., 2016. *Checklist for Autism Friendly Environments.* [Online] Available at: https://positiveaboutautism.co.uk/uploads/9/7/4/5/97454370/checklist_for_autism-friendly_environments_-september_2016.pdf [Accessed 26 10 2021].

Spiers, J., 2019. Introduction. In: E. C. Coalition, ed. *Embracing Complexity: Towards New Approaches for Supporting People with Neurodevelopmental Conditions.* London: Autistica, p. 8.

Standards & Testing Agency, 2020. *The Engagement Model: Guidance for Maintained Schools, Academies (Including Free Schools) and Local Authorities.* [Online] Available at: https://www.gov .uk/government/publications/the-engagement-model [Accessed 19 05 2022].

Webster, A., 2016. *Autism, Sport & Physical Activity.* [Online] Available at: https://england-athletics -prod-assets-bucket.s3.amazonaws.com/2018/11/National-Autism-Society-Autism-sport -physical-activity-PDF-2.1MB-.pdf [Accessed 25 10 2022].

# COMMUNICATION

DOI: 10.4324/9781003154334-7

**Key points**

The National Institute for Health and Care Excellence (NICE) guidelines on the management and support of children and young people on the autism spectrum recommend that
social communication intervention should:

- Be appropriate to the child or young person's developmental level.
- Work towards increasing the parents', carers', teachers' and peers' understanding of
  and sensitivity and responsiveness to the child or young person's patterns of communication and interaction.
- Use therapist modelling and video-interaction feedback.
- Support the development of the child or young person's communication, interactive play and social routines. (National Institute for Health and Care Excellence,
  2021)

Additional important considerations:
- Have a positive attitude towards neurodiversity and autism. The overall aim is to support the young person to advocate for themselves and to listen to **what they identify
  that they do (and do not) need**.
- Consider the impact of the double empathy problem on any communication difficulties.
- Working with the people who are with the child most of the time will support language
  and communication in natural settings.
- Virtual therapy is flourishing and provides real opportunities to work with children and
  young people in alternative environments.

---

Double empathy problem: where there is a communication difficulty, consider how
autistic and neurotypical people understand and respond to each other. There may be
a lack of empathy/understanding in both directions. **Blame for communication breakdown must not be attributed to the autistic young person.**

---

**Areas to consider**
- Support developing autonomy (with appropriate support).
- Consider relationships between the child/young person and significant people in their
  life (e.g. parent/carer/teacher/teaching assistant/siblings/peers). These may not look
  like other (neurotypical) relationships. Opportunity to "be with" other person in emo-
  tionally tuned in social interaction.

- Consider the child/young person's joint/social attention.

- Develop symbolic communication if necessary: single words (any means: speech, symbols, signs) → linking words, particularly verbs and people's names, for a range of purposes, both functional and social.

- Consider narrative and higher language skills (e.g. ability to explain, problem solve, negotiate and justify).

- Consider conversation, which may be different to neurotypical.

- Alongside: consider developing social awareness and understanding (perspective-taking) of the young person and that of their community (mutual understanding).

- Consider play and leisure opportunities, including opportunities to explore autistic identity and develop peer groups.

## Introduction

The communication needs of autistic children and young people will vary from highly articulate to pre-intentional. Within an individual, the communication profile can be "spiky" so that an individual may have strengths and needs, which may vary depending on the setting.

Assessment will clarify if support is needed with *means* to express self and/or with *reasons* or *opportunities*.

Difficulties can be in any or all areas. Support needs to be in place across the child/young person's week through person support (including how people adapt their communication

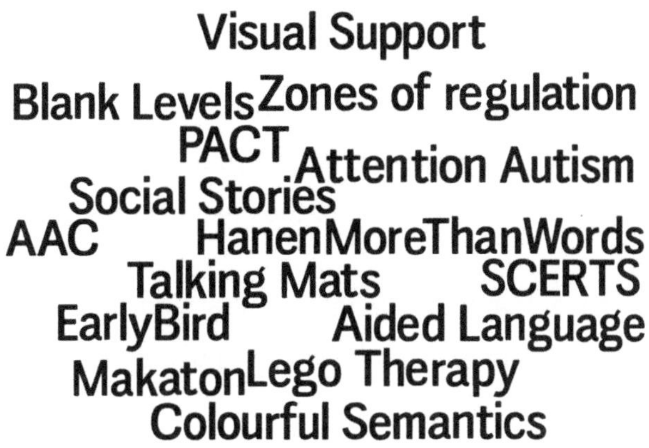

FIGURE 5.1 A selection of interventions used by SLTs.

and interaction style and differentiate expectations) and environmental support (e.g. how the situation is organised).

Chapter 4 focused on environment support. This chapter focuses on support for the child/young person.

## Person support

Several research-based programmes support parents and carers working with autistic children. Following training, the therapist delivers intervention through parent workshops and/or direct work with the child at home or in their educational setting. It is recommended that parent-mediated intervention programmes are considered for parents and carers of all children and young people with autism due to the potential benefits to the child and parent (Scottish Intercollegiate Guidelines Network [SIGN], 2016). Virtual delivery of intervention is gathering a significant and positive evidence base (e.g. Garnett et al., 2022).

These programmes each have their own terminology and strategies.

## Rapport: develop relationships

### Develop skills of communication partners

**Adult's role: priority for all children and young people, whatever their ability: provide opportunities to develop the relationship.**

Autistic children and young people will have differences in social communication, which may need support. An articulate autistic young person could have developed excellent language skills, using them for various purposes. These expressive language skills may mask difficulties with social communication and social understanding. Some youngsters (e.g. many autistic girls) are exceptionally skilled at fitting into social situations, but this comes at a cost to their energy and mental health. These youngsters must have opportunities to relate to others on their terms, which may not look like neurotypical interactions.

Other youngsters will have significant language, learning and/or social communication needs that impact their ability to express themselves using conventional means.

There is good evidence for using video-mediated approaches to support communication development. The National Institute for Health and Care Excellence (NICE) guidelines specifically recommend video-interaction feedback for supporting autistic children and young people (National Institute for Health and Care Excellence, 2021).

Several good practice/evidence-based formal approaches use video effectively to support early communication as part of the programme, including:

- Paediatric autism communication therapy (PACT) uses video feedback with parents/carers in intervention for young children with social communication and language needs associated with autism (Green et al., 2010; Pickles et al., 2016).
- Hanen's More than Words® programme uses video to support the implementation of responsive interaction strategies (www.hanen.org) (Carter et al., 2011).
- The National Autistic Society's EarlyBird programme (autism.org.uk).

## Intensive interaction

Intensive interaction uses video to support the adult in developing their communication skills with a child or young person who may (or may not) be at a very early stage of communication development. It develops the fundamentals of communication through playful, relaxed interactions where the adult responds gently to the young person (Nind & Hewett, 2003).

*What to do*

- Observe the young person.
- Join them.
- Use the communication partner's positioning to support the possibility of interaction: consider being at or below their eye level, within their visual range and their preference (face to face, to the side).
- Give the young person time, no pressure; they take the lead.
- Follow the young person's lead and consider opportunities to join in with an action or sound that the youngster offers.
- Use a minimalist approach.

If actions appear to serve a regulating function, the communication partner should not copy/join in with that aspect of the interaction. Consider their need to regulate. What in the environment contributes to their (lack of) regulation? Consider opportunities for interaction in an optimal environmental situation for the young person.

Use video to reflect on the interaction and the development of the communication partner's skills in following the child/young person's lead.

Seek additional training and supervision to develop skills. The Intensive Interaction Institute website has videos of intensive interaction and further information

www.intensiveinteraction.org.

## Rationale for intensive interaction with more communicative youngsters

Having autism means that the young person will have social communication differences. Following the young person's lead, using their interests, times and places when they are confident, and activities that are familiar and undemanding allow them to focus on the social aspects of the interaction and provide an opportunity to notice, practice and rehearse this. This may feel highly repetitive to the communicative partner. However, the familiarity and safety of the topic and situation provide the opportunity to have a positive social interaction experience, develop rapport and develop skills and/ or confidence in non-verbal aspects of communication if needed/desired. This benefits participation, social understanding and emotional regulation (Mourière & Hewett, 2021; Mouriére, 2018).

Autistic children and young people may have had years of negative responses to their social overtures, contributing to masking, avoidance and trauma (see Chapter 8). Developing positive relationships with a range of people will be the foundation for building trust and identifying a balance between having a comfortable level of support, participation and wellbeing.

## Special Time

For more communicative children and young people encouraging Special Time can benefit building relationships and communication.

Special Time is a planned, consistent time when parent/carer and child play together **without interruptions.** No TV or screens. The child/young person chooses the activity, and you join in. It is not an opportunity to teach or lead. Unless the activity or behaviour is unsafe, do not restrict it.

For the 10 minutes the child is the special focus. No phone calls, conversations with other people, checking email or other distractions are allowed. The child might need some suggestions to get started: play with toys, play a game (hide and seek), make something together (a den), explore something/somewhere (box of toys that have not been looked at for ages).

For young children (up to about seven years): 10 minutes playing daily is ideal.

For older children (about 7–12 years): depending on their attention/developmental level, either 10 minutes a day or 30 minutes a week is excellent.

Teenagers: aim to share an irresistible activity regularly.

*What to do*

- Tune in to the young person: what they do, where they are looking, how they are moving, what they are attending to. Allow plenty of time for interaction.
- Join in with this. Look at their focus of attention and respond to any movements or vocalisation.
- Enjoy this interaction/shared experience.
  This is the foundation to develop the relationship, leading to the development of the young person's skills. It is always on the child/young person's terms. **The adult follows the young person's lead. This gives the young person the opportunity to develop their skills.**

  **Using video allows reflection and development of our/the adult's skills and monitoring of the individual's progress.** Telepractice is being used effectively to support these approaches.

Consider accessing training, e.g.

Intensive Interaction Institute: www.intensiveinteraction.org.

Hanen: www.hanen.org.

PACT: www.pacttraining.co.uk

---

**MAGIC MOMENTS**

Working with people is often challenging, whatever the context. Capturing the magic moments is vital:

- When a magic moment happens, we can be sure that both (all) participants have experienced a positive feeling. This gives a sense of connection.
- It is a positive feeling that participants want to recreate.
- Learning will occur when things have come together in a magic moment (for all participants), although not necessarily the learning you expected.

Teaching skills likely to provide more magic moments to carers is a crucial investment for all.

Tim was an autistic ten-year-old. His anxiety impacted the whole family. On holiday, he expressed his anxiety with repetitive language about his interest: alligators. This caused a great deal of tension as the topic became overwhelming. After a couple of stressful days for everyone, his mother introduced "alli hour," her holiday variant of Special Time. She jotted down a broad plan for the day (e.g. breakfast – swimming pool – lunch – swimming pool – alli hour – eat – bed). She told Tim that in "alli hour" they could play alligator games, talk about 'gators, exchange facts, read his 'gator books and so on. For the rest of the time they would chat about other things. Tim accepted this immediately. Knowing what was happening reduced his anxiety about being on holiday, and knowing that he would get his alligator time transformed the rest of the holiday. Tim loved his "alli hour" and enjoyed the protected time interacting with his mother about his interest. Mum could enjoy the interaction, acknowledging and enjoying Tim's specialist knowledge and sharing the time with him. The whole family benefited from his reduced anxiety and wider opportunities for activities and experiences.

## Attention

**Autistic children and young people often have exceptional attention to their own interests. The people in their environment may not appreciate this if their interests are not valued or the way they express their attention is not recognised.**

Attention deficit (hyperactivity) disorder (ADHD) is associated with autism for many young people; 30–80% of autistic children meet the criteria for ADHD (Rommelse et al., 2010). However, it is vital to consider the role of anxious or agitated behaviour, which may look like ADHD (e.g. restlessness, hypervigilance and increased sensory seeking behaviours).

Task interest, demand and complexity, number of people present and background activity will impact attention.

Teachers of young children in a busy classroom know that they have to actively support pupils to switch attention. Teachers often teach a non-verbal signal (e.g. hands up or a special clap) so that pupils know they must stop an activity, be quiet and listen to the adult. In a busy, noisy classroom with lots of social demands, switching attention is more challenging than in a quiet place with fewer people.

## Active listening

Autistic children and young people may be listening effectively while <u>not</u> demonstrating active listening skills in a typical way. **For many autistic youngsters, being made to look at the person speaking can interfere with their ability to listen effectively. Sitting still may not be indicative of good listening.** Cultural differences in eye gaze also exist, so some communities would not expect their young people to look at the speaker. Using eye contact with an adult, where there is a hierarchy (e.g. teacher–pupil, child–elder), may be considered disrespectful. While many children and young people may quickly and instinctively learn different expectations in different settings, an autistic youngster is likely to find this much more challenging. It may put them at risk of their behaviour or intentions being misunderstood.

> A neurodivergent young person may be paying attention <u>and</u> looking out the window, fiddling with their watch, tapping their feet, searching for their twiddle and humming.

*What to do*

- Be aware of the young person's attention level.
- Develop the team's skills to put supports in place: personal and environmental supports.
- Give the adults/staff clear information about the young person's perspective to support mutual understanding.

Although autistic children do not follow the same developmental path as neurotypical children, awareness of developmental steps can help support understanding of needs and plan support (Table 5.1).

Consider a young person's:

- Attention to objects.
- Attention to other people: face, body language, voice, young person's own name.

*Supporting attention: what to do*

Use the young person's interests to support attention. For example, support the team to

- Use the youngster's interests to support the curriculum (e.g. using counting resources that relate to their interests, reading comprehension of interest).
- Show on schedule access to preferred activities (e.g. science, then... hippo time).
- Some pupils may benefit from knowing the amount of time on an activity; this may be unhelpful for others.

**TABLE 5.1** Attention levels

| Integrated | |
|---|---|
| **Two channelled:** *Can listen whilst doing an activity* <br><br> Consider the next steps: <br><br> ***Practise switching attention.*** <br> ***Attending in more challenging situations*** | *An autistic child/young person's attention may not look like a neurotypical young person's.* **Consider monotropism.** |
| **Single channelled:** *Able to attend to another person's activity with some support.* <br><br> Consider the next step: <br> ***Support young person to learn to switch attention.*** <br> "    "    "    "   ***sustain attention*** to interaction. | |
| **Rigid:** *Able to sustain attention to the preferred activity.* <br><br> Consider the next step: <br> ***Support young person to learn to respond*** to another person's bid for attention. <br><br> ***Support to learn to sustain attention*** (Intensive Interaction, Attention Autism) | |
| **Fleeting:** *May attend to the main stimulus (near, big or emotionally most important stimulus)* <br><br> Consider the next step: <br> ***Support young person to initiate a bid for interaction.*** <br> ***Support adults to follow young person's lead*** (e.g. Intensive Interaction). See Rapport section <br><br> Levels based on (Cooper, et al., 1978) | |

- Support schools to implement flexible break times which reflect the pupils' interests so that the break is a proper break for them and not a social overload. This will support attention when they are in class (e.g. may be appropriate to provide a quiet area with preferred resources away from a busy/noisy playground/classroom to allow a break from the social/sensory demands of school).

Person supports:

- Use the child/young person's name at the start of the interaction.
- Use voice (intonation, stress, volume) to attract and keep attention.
- KISS: keep it (language) short and simple.

Environment supports:

- Control (reduce) background noise (e.g. at home, TV/radio off when focusing on something else).
- Support understanding of routines: timetable, now/next.

Supporting attention in the classroom:

- In class, encourage the use of strategies (e.g. teach and use an agreed signal to gain attention: bell, hand up, clap).

- Give clear (realistic) expectations of attention and feedback.
- AND make reasonable adjustments for autistic child/young person (and other neuro-divergent youngsters):
    - Consider providing a distinct space (e.g. mat, hoop, bobbly cushion) and positioning preference (e.g. back to the wall, near adult, in the middle of the group, at the front for the best view, at the back so that the pupil can see what is going on around them, at the edge to give space for some movement without disrupting peers).
    - Consider sensory needs (sitting on a chair versus the floor, textured/firm/unstable surface, with foot/back support, allow for movement), noise (ear defenders/noise cancelling headphones), control/warning of change to volume, lighting, etc. Allow for movement.
    - Provide planned movement breaks if needed.
    - Learning breaks.
    - Allow (promote) fiddles. Make adjustments if necessary to accommodate.
    - Promote adequate water/hydration.

Typical "good listening rules" that might be used in a mainstream primary classroom may need significant reasonable adjustment for an autistic child or young person:

- Looking at the eyes of the person talking may be highly uncomfortable, so the young-ster **may not be able to** look at the speaker and concentrate/listen.
- Consider sensory needs: an autistic child/young person sitting still may not indicate good attention (e.g. may be frozen in fright mode). Consider positioning and providing an opportunity for safe movement with advice from an occupational therapist if appropriate.

These are to support the young person's understanding of the routine, NOT to enforce compliance. Times may OR MAY NOT be helpful for the individual.

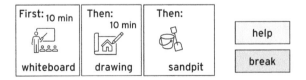

Clock with hour hand and symbols can support understanding of day as an alternative to timetable:

**FIGURE 5.2** Environmental supports: to help understanding/attention.

## Joint attention

**Joint attention** is where two (or more) people share a focus on an object or activity, and they are aware of the shared interest. This is fundamental to the development of social communication and would usually be established by 18 months. Joint attention is seen in eye gaze (accompanied by pointing in many cultures) to share interest in an item. Noticing someone looking at an object, at you, then back at the object and looking there is one way that joint attention is demonstrated: using eye gaze to look between a person's face and object. In an autistic child/young person, joint attention may be displayed differently or may not be observed.

Joint attention and social interest are typically expressed non-verbally in young children. Pointing and eye contact are conventional ways of expression. Pointing and eye gaze differences should be discussed with the family to determine whether the observed behaviours are appropriate. For example, how do they compare to siblings and other children in the community, which may not be the same as expected within the therapist's community?

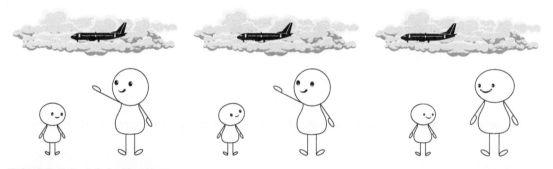

**FIGURE 5.3** Joint attention.

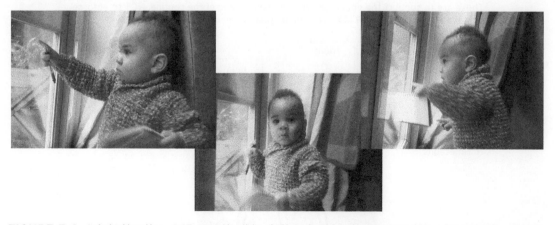

**FIGURE 5.4** Joint attention. A 15-month-old pointing, looking to carer and then back to the object.

Language without joint attention:

Karl was standing in his empty classroom with his coat, saying, "Help, please." He had the linguistic skill to ask for help but did not direct his request to someone who could help him.

Joint attention without language:

Laura looked at her mum, showed her a ball and looked back at her mum's face to check what she had seen. She lacked the linguistic skill to make a request using language, but she could express that she wanted the ball pool.

An autistic child may express interest **differently** from a neurotypical child (Jaswala & Akhtarb, 2019). They may focus less on people and more on objects, particularly on their interests. Their attention could be excellent, but social/joint attention may need to be established. This can be supported using relationship-based approaches (e.g. Intensive Interation), which focus on the young person's interests.

The development of joint attention supports learning. For example:

- Supporting attention to language learning.
- Developing non-verbal skills/social communication.
- Can support awareness of "hidden communication."

A child may be highly focused on a computer game and appear immersed, not offering obvious cues for social engagement (e.g. not showing the screen, pointing to an item of interest, commenting to another person or looking between the screen and another person). Still, despite this lack of shared interest (from a neurotypical perspective), the child could be engaging socially by playing with a peer online, noticing someone commenting enthusiastically on the activity and responding and imitating another person's action within the game. They might converse about the game with another "expert" gamer in extended conversational turns, which could be described as "monologues" by a neurotypical outsider, but accepted as chat by their autistic peer. Their conversational turns may be much longer, persistence to the same topic considered relevant and interesting, and ending the conversation abruptly unremarkable.

## Resources and activities

*Responding to joint attention*

**What's in the bag?** An adult has a bag or box of resources that appeal to the child(ren)/ young person. This might include items that are interesting visually or audibly. These are introduced one at a time in a predictable, repetitive way. Both the item and the adult's presentation are engaging to the youngster. Communication skills are modelled. Watch, listen and give plenty of time to provide the child/young person with the opportunity to respond to the item/person. All communication is accepted and validated; it may be modelled (e.g. a sign attempt copied to demonstrate the sign clearly) and extended.

All of these can be used to support the development of joint attention, with the child watching the adult doing the activity (attention or two-way attention: child looking at the activity), leading to looking between the person and the activity (joint attention or three-way attention: child looking between activity and person).

*What to do*

- Choose something from the bag.
- Use a predictable routine. Consider using a short, memorable song or rhyme and action.
- Introduce the item and show it near your face.
- Use proximity, facial expression, body language and eye gaze carefully.
- Use language and vocalisation with great care. Consider your use of volume and intonation. Focus on core vocabulary: useful words that can be used in many situations (go, more, look, finished, like, stop). Say little, for a specific reason and give plenty of time to process and respond.
- Use pauses to allow time to process and respond.
- Repeat two or three times.

If working in a small group, give any adults guidance on their role to support the pupils: be excellent role models.

Look for:
- Gestures: reaching, pointing, give me, show.
- Eye gaze: looking between object and person (adult leading activity and carer if present). Eye contact is not necessary.
- Proximity.

- Vocalisation.
- Facial expression.
- Body language.

Notice the child/young person's wellbeing/enjoyment.

Gina Davies has developed practical and fun approaches using techniques that are particularly helpful in teaching attention, communication and social interaction skills: the Curiosity Programme™ and Attention Autism™ (Davies, 2022). An underlying principle is that engaging the child by offering an irresistible invitation to learn is the first critical step to success.

**The Curiosity Programme**™ breaks down the stages needed to develop an individual's skills if they are not ready for the group approach to Attention Autism™. This initially uses shared exploration (watching how the young person explores a preferred resource, joining in and enjoying the interaction), gradually imposing more curiosity and interaction, adding rhymes/songs to routines, exploratory play and playing together to build skills.

**Attention Autism**™ uses four stages within a small group. This develops attention, communication and social interaction by building on attention skills from early joint attention. Children learn to attend to an activity designed to be engaging by using sensory activities, often using visually attractive resources, sustaining this attention and developing and building on skills to switch attention and sustain attention independently within an activity.

This approach can be adapted to fit with curriculum areas in early years and school settings and to support the development of independence skills. It starts by using activities designed to be appealing to the participants to capture and then sustain attention and encourage communication in response to the activity. The activities become more goal orientated through the programme so that the children/young people follow the other person's agenda, sustaining and eventually switching attention independently.

Activities can be linked to curriculum areas as children and young people move into and through school to support engagement in topics using the approach as a whole, or using it for starter and/or plenary activities.

Activities throughout the day to develop awareness/response to joint/social attention:

- Interaction games/songs/routines: for younger children, interactive songs (Row the Boat, Round and Round the Garden, Walk along Josie), older children/young people may have interaction routines specific to particular individuals. Support may be needed (with language or social demands) to develop these, particularly in less familiar settings or with unfamiliar people. Using interests may be helpful, although the young person's knowledge and skills are likely to be far superior to their communication partner, so their motivation to attend to an unskilled partner may be limited!

- Unexpected event that the young person notices (e.g. tower of building blocks falls, low flying plane, spillage), "oops" and look between the child's face and the object.
- Hide and seek: "find" the child/young person's preferred objects around the room.
  - Use a reach/contact point (e.g. touch item) and look at their face as you find it.
  - Gradually fade to a distant (distal) point (where the item is out of reach).
  - Fade point to look at the item.
- Awareness of hidden communication: in a (very) small group, throw a bean bag/squishy ball:
  - Say the child's name and then throw a ball/bean bag to them, and they throw it back.
  - Look to the child and throw to the child/young person (scaffold with body language, gradually reduce clues until the child responds to you looking).
- Awareness of hidden communication: wink murder (or sleep game): youngsters take turns identifying who is sending everyone to sleep. Starting with a gesture, an obvious nod, fading to a blink, then reducing clues to a subtle wink.
- Changing places: small group sits in a circle with one empty chair.
  - Start using the youngster's name to choose who will move to the empty chair.
  - Move on to a look and point, gradually fade to using only eye gaze to look towards (eye contact not necessary), and that person moves to the empty chair (just following gaze, awareness of hidden communication).
  - Eventually play so that the person who moves to the empty chair becomes the leader and chooses the next person to move so that people are watching more faces.
  - Add another empty chair and direct the person where to sit non-verbally "who" are you addressing? "where" should they sit? Participants choose how they will direct each other.

The purpose is <u>not</u> to improve eye contact, which would harm many autistic young people, but to increase awareness of the hidden social clues of communication. The games increase awareness, and opportunities for discussion about real-life social clues should be prioritised to support perspective-taking (see section titled "Social understanding").

## Play

Play facilitates the development of social communication skills, including turn-taking, sharing, collaborating, negotiating, reciprocating and developing friendships.

Autistic children and young people may not follow a typical developmental sequence for play. For example:

- Sensorimotor activities may be necessary for self-regulation (e.g. comfort/calming) and may be used more than expected.
- The young person may have more advanced skills in some areas (e.g. highly skilled in construction or IT).
- Incorporating ideas from peers and imaginative play with peers are likely to be challenging.
- The young person may have different play preferences (e.g. organising toys by size, lining up, preference for sensory play and complex role-playing games).

The diversity of play in autistic children and young people will depend on their cognitive and linguistic abilities. The diversity in play reflects the diversity of autism (Kossyvaki & Papoudi, 2016).

## What to do

Consider:

- Developmental (play) level of the young person.
- Their interests.
- Adult support/involvement/guided play/"authentic" peers.
- Naturalistic development approaches.

**Exploratory play**: offer plenty of opportunities for play with various objects and toys that provide a variety of multisensory experiences. Ensure that these are safe (non-toxic, no small parts that are detachable by a curious young person) and that the child/young person is supervised. The child/young person gets the opportunity to explore play materials, an adult playing with or alongside the child.

Watch. Join in and copy the child's play. Observe the child's awareness of your involvement and consider extending play slightly OR intruding slightly into their play (e.g. taking a turn in an activity, perhaps with a slightly different action, or holding a resource back and pausing).

**Resources:** bubbles, foam, dough, slime, musical instruments, bricks, construction toys, sand, paint (including clean messy play where messy resources are bagged into tough sealed plastic bags), pompoms, ribbons, balloons (blown up and tied, blown up and tied with rice inside, blow and release, with helicopter, car, whistle attachments, containing foam, confetti, lights), sensory balls, wind-up toys, pop-up toys, sensory bottles or bags, sand, water, etc.

**TABLE 5.2** Neurotypical play

| *Play* | *Social play* |
|---|---|
| **Exploratory play**<br>Sensory exploration → object exploration:<br>Repeating movements:<br>• Moving body: arms, hands, legs, feet.<br>• Shaking rattles, banging items. Items often mouthed. | **Solitary**<br>But interaction/play with caregivers for bonding (smiling, gazing, blinking, sticking out tongue, vocalising).<br>Reliant on caregiver following infant's lead. |
| **Relational play**<br>• Functional: cause–effect play (push buttons, turn handles, pop-up toys, throw, put toys together, knock them down).<br>• Imitative: copy the caregiver stirring a drink.<br>• Relational: pushing a car, blowing a balloon.<br><br>**Gross motor play:** running, swinging, climbing. | Mostly solitary but more responsive to caregivers. Play with caregivers provides an opportunity to practice some early social games: e.g. chase, hide and seek, ball games. |
| **Pretend/symbolic play**<br>• The child pretends to sleep, to have a drink, says "moo" when playing with pretend cow, etc.<br>• Pretend directed to others (often eating and self-care routines initially), then using unrealistic or pretend objects to stand in for something in play (banana telephone, pretend a drink is hot).<br>• Linking symbolic play sequences: feeding dolly and putting to bed. Getting on the train and going to the seaside.<br>• Dolly/action figure becomes active, taking the lead.<br>• Substitutions for missing items used imaginatively. | **Onlooker/spectator**<br>Watch peers, but not join in.<br><br>**Parallel play**<br>Playing alongside others, but not with peers. |
| **Construction (fine motor)**, puzzles, drawing.<br>• Table games: e.g. snap, snakes and ladders, Game of Life, Risk, draughts, chess, role play.<br>• Screen games. | **Associative play**<br>Share resources, playing on the same equipment, but not playing together. |
| **Complex play**<br>• Complex stories acted out with toys or role played socially: face to face or virtually. | **Cooperative play**<br>Working together to achieve a shared outcome, interested in the activity and other children. |

Social media groups (YouTube, Facebook groups, Pinterest, etc.) have endless sugges-tions for effective play options, from simple, quick and clean through to more special-ist and complex ideas (e.g. slime recipes avoiding particular ingredients, helpful for young people with allergies/sensitivities or who need edible recipes).

The child/young person may want to explore items through tapping, banging, mouthing, biting and throwing as well as more conventional play.

Watch the child/young person; the child takes the lead, give them plenty of time and join the child in their play; 80% at the child's current level, 20% extend (e.g. through demonstration/modelling).

Consider the purpose of your involvement in the child/young person's play. For example:

- Developing relationships: join in, minimalistic approach, non-directive.
- Developing play: join in, the child takes the lead, consider extending/intruding slightly (80:20).
- Developing language: modelling language, aided language support (see chapter 9).

**Relational play (cause-effect)** allows the young person to learn about cause and effect: their actions and their impact on the world around them. This can include toy play and person play. Toy play might have sound, movement, visual interest or a construction ele-ment: e.g. fitting together or opening/closing. Person play will include familiar play rou-tines ("ready, steady... go" games knocking down towers, blowing bubbles, ball runs, rolling cars, blowing up and releasing balloons, etc., "come to me" running into caregiver's arms for a twirl, tickles or a hug, etc.).

**Resources:** cause-effect toys, for example: balloons/spinners/pop-up toys/car or ball runs/squeaky toys/musical toys/light up toys/containers/shape sorters/stacking toys/ pop-up books/boxes/bags/purses.

Unexpected play

No play should be considered entirely inappropriate, although it may not be an ideal place or time for a particular type of activity. For example, spitting is appropriate in teeth cleaning, kicking when playing football and biting when eating. When activities are unsafe, look for the consequences for the child or young person. For example, are they getting adult <u>attention,</u> <u>avoiding</u> an activity or achieving <u>sensory</u> feedback supporting emotional regulation?

## Pretend/symbolic play

Pretend play helps develop a young person's symbolic understanding needed for language development.

Consider having two sets of resources of interest to the young person. These could be identical or a mixture of matched and complementary toys (e.g. one person has a train, and the other has a track) suitable for pretend play.

Incorporate play opportunities within the curriculum:

- Use characters and resources from a story (e.g. English, humanities) and provide opportunities for play, e.g. Three Little Pigs, War Horse. Small-world play might involve toy animals and materials. Role play might involve masks and larger resources: straws, sticks and boxes to make buildings. Both could be used to develop their play or re-enact the story playfully.
- Use resources in other curriculum areas and give opportunities for exploratory and pretend play (e.g. science - playing scientists: doctors, astronauts, geologists, palaeontologists, etc.; maths - cutting pretend pizzas and sharing out, sorting items by different criteria playfully).

A recent review of research to identify the best intervention for play for autistic children and young people identified common themes:

- Consider the child's developmental level and interests.
- Consider using:
  - Guided play: a prepared environment with adult scaffolding.
  - Adult support and involvement during play.
  - Involvement of authentic peers.
- The likely value of naturalistic developmental approaches: using incidental learning opportunities to support development through carefully planned support to help scaffold the next step to develop skills (O'Keeffe & McNally, 2021).

*What to do*

- Use the young person's interests. **Allow plenty of opportunities for the child/young person to play on their own terms, in their own way.**
- Follow their lead:
  - Watch what the young person is doing.
  - Listen.
  - Consider the purpose of your intervention. Ensure the child has plenty of opportunities to play independently.
  - Join in: consider offering opportunities: **copying**, **responding to** or **extending** their play. Extending can mean:
    - Offering new resources within the same play themes.
    - Providing opportunities for the same play in a new setting.
    - Introducing the same play alongside/with new person/people.
    - Introducing new ideas to the same resources.

> Playtime or break time should be when the child/young person can have a break from (learning) demands. If this is used as a learning opportunity for a youngster, then it is vital to ensure that they have an opportunity to have a break when they can engage in their own choice of activity without imposing social or other demands in an environment that is acceptable.

## Social communication with peers

Some autistic children and young people relate well to adults. They are articulate, able to use language effectively for a range of reasons and may seek and enjoy interaction with adults. Social communication difficulties may not be evident within a clinical setting, where some youngsters can relate appropriately to an unfamiliar adult. Social expectations are relatively straightforward, and the adult often scaffolds the youngster's interaction. Some autistic children play and interact much better with younger peers. This may be because the social hierarchy is clear: the older child is higher up the hierarchy, but with very young children, they may be able to adapt communication to a style that suits the younger child and so have a successful and mutually enjoyable experience.

As with any individual, an autistic young person may want to spend time with people with similar interests. Research and anecdotal reports show that two autistic participants can be more interactive than an autistic and neurotypical pair. For example, a small study compared a conversation between two autistic participants who did not know each other to a conversation between the autistic person and their neurotypical friend and between the autistic person and an unfamiliar neurotypical person. It was found that in conversations between two autistic participants, the flow, rapport and attunement between partners were significantly increased (Williams et al., 2021). Autistic children and young people must be supported to have opportunities to get to know an autistic peer group.

## Social play

Play can be alone or social (with adults or peers of the same/different age, with/without autism or additional needs).

Peer play can be:

- Free (no adult involvement).
- Guided (adult involved, but led by a child).
- Structured (led by an adult).

The content of play can be an object (e.g. exploratory, sensory), game (snap, snakes and ladders, Connect Four, Uno, draughts, chess), imaginative (small-world play, role play including fantasy role play) or digital (all sorts: duplicates of other play). Virtual play with others can reduce social demands and lead to more social engagement for some young-sters. Playing alongside is enjoyable and fulfilling for some, providing a feeling of connec-tion without being overwhelming (Aut, 2021).

The preferences of the youngster are of particular significance. Use strategies (e.g. Talking Mats) to identify what the child/young person wants in terms of peer interaction: e.g. play, conversation or relationships, and consideration of communication preferences: in real life/face-to-face, synchronous (i.e. "live") communication, via text, email, messaging (asynchronous) communication.

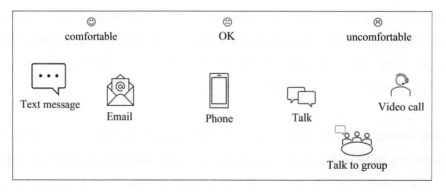

**FIGURE 5.5** Talking Mat: communication preferences.

**Lego®-Based Therapy** (LeGoff et al., 2014) provides engaging, naturalistic learning opportunities to develop language and social communication using a familiar resource, usually using a collaborative framework where there is a "supplier" who finds the bricks, an "engineer" who has the plans and a "builder" who makes the model. The same approach can be used with many different activities, e.g. cooking and crafting.

## Language

Some language and communication differences are associated with autism, and some difficulties occur with autism. These can be as diverse as for any child, although some recurring themes exist. The focus of this section is on differences that are more specific to autistic children and young people.

Differences:

- Need more processing time: this may be due to different language processing styles: single words rather than sentence level (Cullen, 2021) and see Figure 4.5.
- Use of personal pronouns (e.g. I/you) or referring to self by own name.
- Echolalia (gestalt language learning style): immediate and/or delayed echolalia may be used effectively/communicatively.
- Unexpected verbal responses are relatively common. This may be for several reasons, including:
  - Needing more processing time, so responding to a previous question.
  - Focusing on detail (monotropism), so responding to a detail rather than a whole situation.
  - Reduced semantic priming. Usually, when a word is heard or read, the brain primes so that a semantically related word/idea may be expected (e.g. *fish and...* semantic priming means that we expect to hear "chips"). This may be different, so the individual does not get a semantic clue that would be expected, and they do not make the connection that might seem obvious.
- Despite adequate or excellent language skills, some autistic people experience difficulties using language in some situations. They may be *selective in their use of verbal language* (may use augmentative and alternative communication [AAC] in some situations), or they may *rely heavily on preparation*. Situations that rely on fast communication where the content cannot be foreseen (e.g. answering unpredictable questions in a job interview or social chit-chat) may be of no interest or highly challenging.

A "spiky" profile is common, so the young person has strengths in one area but needs support in another. This might seem unexpected in the context of their strengths, leading to unreasonable expectations.

## Echolalia (gestalt language learning style)

Some children and young people learn language in larger units than single words. This is used communicatively for a variety of purposes, for example:

- Acknowledging: verbally acknowledging the other person's language (e.g. the child/young person may not have understood but is socially engaged and repeats to acknowledge).
- Initiating (and sustaining) a familiar interaction routine, e.g. following a script or another person repeats and then the youngster continues: a conversation but without having to generate/process the content. It could be a familiar song/game ("The time has come to say goodnight...," "Round and round the garden..." or a more personal "Monday" *"school and ICT,"* "Tuesday" *"school and swimming...,"* "Saturday" *"home!"* "Sunday" *"home"*).
- Expressing emotion: e.g. "you have caused confusion and delay" to express upset (from Thomas and Friends) or "mummy's at home" expressing anxiety (and probably a request to go home).
- Requesting: "you want water?" (meaning "I want water").

Evidence supports echolalia as an interactive occurrence (Sterponi & Shankey, 2014) and an adaptation to support forming relationships and social-emotional attachments (Stiegler, 2015). This supports interventions that do not attempt to eliminate echolalia, but that focus on:

- Consideration of how echolalia is used.
  - For relationship building/maintenance: playful use of repetitive language.
  - Immediate echolalia: using the same words to express functions (e.g. immediately repeating "do you want milk?" could mean *yes, I want milk*, or could be an acknowledgement of the interaction, but without understanding).
  - Delayed echolalia: using chunks of learned language at another time, which may or may not have a clear function. The reason could be regulatory (the youngster appears highly focused, narrating dialogue from a familiar film in a busy classroom, shutting out overwhelming stimuli) or communicative ("mummy's at home" may be expressing anxiety about school or mum, may be requesting to go home or may be asking when is it home time, "all better now" when child has fallen over and has grazed knee).
  - Echolalia used generatively: may use parts of echolalia and start to use generatively ("I like your nails" changing to "I like your hair," "I like your leggings").

*What to do*

- Develop initiation (e.g. through intensive interaction).
- Consider the interaction style of the communication partner. A focus on "doing with" and responsive communication, considering the non-verbal aspects and function of the interaction rather than a directive, questioning interaction style, is supportive.
- Consider the young person's understanding. Use visual support (objects or pictures/ symbols). Consider a focus on aspects of echolalia (e.g. "I like your hair," "let's go and play") and preferred activities to support understanding of components of language. This allows for playful modelling of generative language.

Consider the use of visual support to continue to develop an understanding and use of language for a range of reasons. For example, in Chapter 2, Lara talked about "I like your hair" and "I like your nails." What started as a single repetitive social starter that served her well in building relationships developed as she learned to manipulate language and extend the interaction. This provided other people with the opportunity to use the familiar form to model with colour-coded visual support:

- I like your shoes.
- Your shoes (are) new/wet.
- Get your shoes.
- Your bag is wet.
- Careful, the nail varnish is wet!
- Your hands are wet.

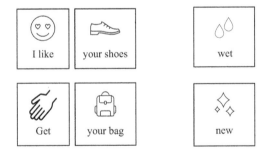

## Understanding spoken language

- Different processing styles impact understanding for many autistic children and young people, thus:
  - Non-literal and ambiguous language is challenging.
  - More processing time may be needed.
  - Context may not be used alongside language, impacting understanding.

In addition, symbolic understanding is challenging for some autistic children and young people, affecting their understanding of spoken language, signing, gestures, etc. Augmentative

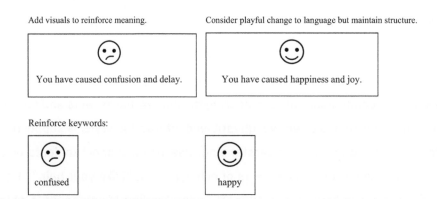

Add visuals to reinforce meaning.

You have caused confusion and delay.

Consider playful change to language but maintain structure.

You have caused happiness and joy.

Reinforce keywords:

confused

happy

**FIGURE 5.6** Supporting generative language.

**TABLE 5.3** Symbolic representation

| Object | Photo | Picture/symbol | Gesture/sign | Spoken word → written word |
|---|---|---|---|---|
| **Representational** (empty travel toothpaste)<br><br>**Miniature** (travel toothbrush)<br><br>**Part** (toothpaste)<br><br>**Complete** (toothbrush/paste in a see-through bag)<br><br>Helpful to have a place to put the item to mark the activity (e.g. toothpaste into a cup by the sink). | **Representational item** (a generic photo)<br><br>**Actual item** (photo of actual item)<br><br>Use photos carefully. A photo of a London bus may be much harder to understand than a picture if the actual bus is a Manchester bus. | **Black and white**<br><br>**Coloured** (colours can be misleading if they do not match reality) | **Makaton**<br><br>**Gesture**<br><br>Youngster's own use of gestures (reach, push, point) | cake ↓ cake |

communication (e.g. visual support: signing, symbols, objects) is relevant to supporting understanding, but not all children and young people benefit from the same type of support.

Children at an early stage of language development typically use many context clues to support their understanding: body language, tone of voice and context. Identifying how useful these are to the autistic young person and then using these to support understanding is extremely helpful. Introducing Makaton signing may help a young person who consistently benefits from gestures. Consideration of formalising situational clues with picture or object support would be helpful (see table 5.4).

## Object of reference

**An object that represents a particular meaning (e.g. an object, activity, place, time).**

Visual information supports understanding, memory and organisation. For some, an object is easier to interpret than an image. It can be seen and handled. The same object is consistently used to mean the same thing.

An object of reference can be:

- A real object (e.g. lunchbox=lunchtime, toilet roll=toilet, swimming costume=swimming).
- Part of a real object (inside of loo roll=toilet, empty bag of crisps = crisps, ribbon from teddy bear=bed).
- A miniature object (toy car=car, toy duck=bath).
- A representational object (specific scarf=grandma).

The item should be given to the child/young person just before the activity and used every time.

The item should be meaningful and motivating: consider the item from the youngsters' perspective (e.g. bus: adult's perspective – bus pass, child's perspective – lanyard they might play with on the bus; bath: adult's perspective – soap or sponge, child's perspective – bath toy). Be aware that objects might not be the same in different situations (e.g. family use loo rolls at home, but these may not be used in school). Object associations can be taught if these are not already clear (e.g. using a scarf to represent a particular person).

Using a "construction" approach where the child puts two items together can be helpful (toilet: loo roll on loo roll holder; tabletop activity: puzzle piece into the puzzle on the table; soft play: ball into the ball pool; cooking: wooden spoon into utensil drawer or pot; playtime: hoop on the post in the playground; home time: water bottle into bag).

Objects of reference:

- Help the young person's understanding: give the item to the youngster as you say the word. Allow them to handle the object, and give them time to explore.
- Support memory: the object stays and speech disappears once the word has been said.
- Help with transitions: tell the individual what is happening as you give the item. Objects of reference can be used in a timetable (e.g. using hanging shoe storage).
- Help making choices (e.g. art [paintbrush] or cooking [wooden spoon]).
- Help making requests: for items, for activities, to go to places.

| Level 1: Naming | Level 3: Retelling |
|---|---|
| What is it?<br>Show me a ...<br>Find one like this...<br>What's this called?<br>What can you see?<br>*What are you touching?*<br>*What can you hear?*<br>*What can you smell?*<br>Say this...<br><br><br>*Italics* are more abstract for most youngsters. | Tell the story.<br>Find one that is... & ...<br>How did they... (make the cake)?<br>What could (s)he say?<br>What will happen next?<br>What else... (flies)?<br>Which one is not... (an animal)?<br>What happened to all of these?<br>How are these the same?<br>What is... (a kettle)? |
| **Level 2: Describing** | **Level 4: Justifying** |
| What is (s)he doing?<br>Tell me the (colour, size, shape).<br>Where is he?<br>Who is in the story?<br>What things... (can fly)?<br>Find one that is...<br>How are these two different?<br>Finish this: I like to eat... / what do you like to…?<br>Find one that can... (cut).<br>What is happening? | Why...?<br>What could (s)he do to solve the problem?<br>How do you know?<br><br>*Warm up at an easier level, then work at the child's current level, model at the next level.*<br>*Step down a level if it is tricky.*<br>*Step up if it is easy.* |

Based on Blank et al., 1978

**FIGURE 5.7** Blank levels bookmark.

Objects can be labelled with a picture or symbol; this may be a stepping-stone to using symbols (without the object).

-----------------------------------------------------------------------------------------

## Blank levels (Blank et al., 1978)

Widely used in Australia and highlighted in the United Kingdom by ELKLAN (Elks & McLachlan, 2009), Blank levels support understanding of spoken language and the child/young person's ability to respond to questions. Knowing a child/young person's Blank level helps make certain that other people use language appropriately to ensure understanding. The youngster's language level can be challenged by modelling language at a higher level. This is extremely helpful in schools where teachers can differentiate by careful use of language and questioning.

Blank levels work extremely well in conjunction with colour-coded picture support. Colour coding helps with understanding and using sentences and particularly helps autistic children and young people who are often relatively strong in understanding and using nouns but may have more difficulty using verbs and proper nouns (people's names) and more abstract language. The *Test of Abstract Language Comprehension* (TALC) and TALC 2 (for secondary/college-aged pupils) (Elks & McLachlan, 2007; McLachlan & Elks, 2010) are straightforward assessments that help identify needs and can be used to monitor progress. *Language for Thinking* (Parsons & Branagan, 2016) also uses Blank levels. Twinkl (Twinkl, 2022) has resources based on Blank levels.

Level 1: naming (nouns). What is it? Point to the (bus)? Get a (pencil).

Level 2: describing (verbs, adjectives, adverbs, etc.). Find a (blue) one. Which one can (swim)? What does it do?

Level 3: retelling, defining, negating.

Level 4: explaining, justifying, negotiating.

The Blank levels bookmark can be used alongside a reading book with the relevant sections highlighted to focus the adult reading with the child on the appropriate language level for the pupil. Reading can include books without words and all kinds of reading material. The same language levels are relevant in other activities: watching and talking about something on TV, cooking together and playing at the park and in school or nursery.

In addition to the Blank level, consider the impact on understanding of:

- Emotional load: understanding where either the situation or topic is anxiety provoking will be harder, and this may not be predictable to the other person.

- The young person's personal experience of the topic.
- Familiarity with vocabulary.
- "Hands on"/"here and now" versus something in the past and/or more abstract.

*What to do*

Check in with the young person, what do they need?

Provide visual supports. Encourage use of day-to-day strategies to support understanding:

- Invite their responses, but be prepared to support understanding/responses by:
  - Having a peer model first.
  - Providing an example.
  - Showing (video/photo/demonstration).

Provide help identifying a lack of understanding and seeking effective support.

- Model lack of understanding, for example:
  - Too quiet.
  - Unfamiliar words.
  - Too much background noise.
  - Too much information.
- Work with the child/young person to identify what they NEED to support understanding:
  - Additional time.
  - Modification of language.
  - Hands-on learning/experience.
  - Demonstration/modelling.

Table 5.4 is a prompt sheet for observing children and young people and considering what might be supporting their understanding. For example, a young person with extremely

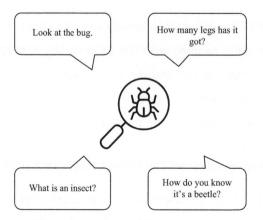

**FIGURE 5.8** Blank levels (science example questions).

**TABLE 5.4** What helps child/young person's understanding of language

Understanding:
Blank level <1, 1, 2, 3, 4
What helps:

- Context (layout/familiarity/routines)
- Personal experience
- Particular interest
- Vocabulary knowledge
- Body language
- Tone of voice
- Social context (copying peers)
- Other visual supports
- Processing time (how long?)
- Concrete – abstract
- Literal – ambiguous
- Differentiation of speaker

limited understanding of spoken language might be reported to "understand everything," but they may be using other strategies:

- Following the routines effectively, e.g. hanging up their coat.
- Following the adult's eye gaze and going to stand by the door ready to go to assembly.
- Sitting on the carpet with the other pupils.
- Using intonation to understand when a teacher is asking a question and making a response.

## Expressive language

There is a considerable variation in expressive language ability. The aspiration for all children and young people is to have the means to be able to communicate for a wide range of reasons (Figure 5.9), using any means of communication. Ensuring that the young person is supported to develop appropriate means of communicating for a wide range of reasons that are listened to will contribute to wellbeing. Without effective strategies for refusal, protest, negotiation and expression of emotions, the young person is likely to develop unhelpful methods to communicate these functions. This will result in either loss of participation due to withdrawal as they opt out or loss of opportunity as they are considered unable to participate in the situation in a way that is considered socially appropriate.

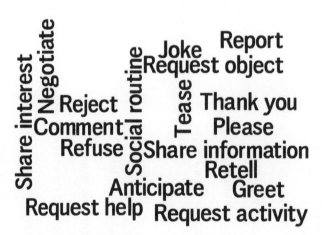

FIGURE 5.9 Reasons for communicating.

**Pre-intentional:** child/young person may (appear to) have limited means and/or reasons to communicate.

At this stage, the young person focuses on their needs, interests and activities. Other people recognise their needs, desires and interests through observation of behaviour rather than conventional communication. For example, noticing the youngster's activity, their focus of attention, facial expression or crying.

***Essential for all:*** rapport/being with other people (see section titled "Rapport: develop relationships")/emotional regulation (see Chapter 6).

- Support adults in the young person's environment to follow their lead and develop the relationship. Develop the communication partner's responsiveness to the individual (noticing and responding to their non-verbal communication). Copy with care.
- Increase the young person's ability to initiate interaction and then sustain the exchange (the adult following the young person's lead).

These opportunities can be through timetabled sessions and incidental learning moments throughout the day.

**Intentional (non-verbal):** may have limited means or reasons to communicate.

At this stage, the young person is developing an awareness of other people and may be expressing intentions, such as wants and/or protests. This may be through any means (e.g. reaching or pushing).

*Important for all*: rapport/being with other people/emotional regulation (Chapter 6)/joint attention/anticipating/requesting using more conventional means.

Develop the young person's autonomy:

- Ability of the people around them to provide an environment that promotes responsive, social interaction so that they can initiate social interaction (not just interaction to meet wants/needs).
- Ability of the people around them to provide an environment with many opportunities to communicate.
- Ability of the child/young person to express themselves so they can request an item or activity using eye gaze, reach, vocalisation/word, point (contact and distance).

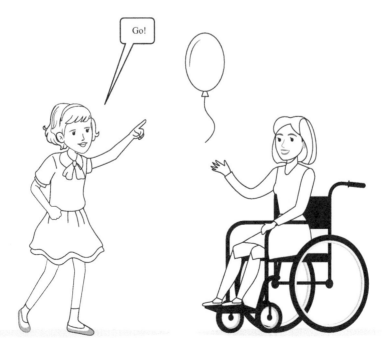

**FIGURE 5.10** Using anticipation to support first words.

Encourage appealing activities with lots of communication opportunities (see sections titled "Attention" and "Play").

- Ability to express a choice, initially using reach, give and point gestures to choose from two objects.

Activities that support attention and play are often effective in developing first words using anticipation, pause and modelling, as used in Hanen's More Than Words (Sussman, 2012), PACT and EarlyBird approaches. Supporting carers to follow the child's lead, develop the interaction through using the child's interests, gently joining in and developing opportunities to interact alongside careful use of language (e.g. commenting occasionally on what the child is doing) lead to an increase in initiation and responding (Garnett et al., 2022).

More explicit teaching is needed for some children and young people. PECS® (Pyramid Educational Consultants®, n.d.) uses a highly structured protocol to teach functional communication using picture exchange. Objects can be exchanged instead of symbols to make a request, which is helpful for youngsters at a very early stage of symbolic understanding or with visual difficulties.

An adaptation uses a box exchange to teach the individual to make an exchange for an item that they want, which often avoids the need for a physical prompt. The child passes a transparent box containing the item they want to the adult. The box has a picture of the desired item on it. After successful exchanges, the child can learn to exchange the picture rather than the box, introducing symbolic understanding. **This is a stepping-stone to support the development of symbolic understanding so the child/young person can start communicating about items they cannot see.** A picture is a more concrete symbol than a spoken word, supporting the development of symbolic representation.

- Enticing activities are used to engage the young person.
- Activities can be tangible, sensory and social.
- It helps if activities have a natural endpoint so that individuals get the opportunity to request again.
- Real situations can be used with actual activities in natural settings.
- Minimal language is involved.
- Motivation comes from the youngster as the activities appeal to their interests.

A core vocabulary, useful words that can be helpful in all contexts alongside vocabulary usually expected in early communication development, e.g. from communication development inventories (Alcock et al., 2020), provides a range of means for communication. See Chapter 9 for more information about using a core vocabulary (AAC) approach.

# First words

At this stage, young people use single words (including AAC) to express themselves.

*Important for all*: being with other people/emotional regulation (see Chapter 6)/joint attention/anticipating/requesting/protesting/refusing using more conventional means/using language for a range of purposes.

Develop the young person's autonomy:

- Ability of the people around them to provide an environment that promotes responsive, social interaction so that they can initiate social interaction (not just interaction to meet wants/needs).
- Ability of people around them to provide an environment with lots of opportunities to communicate.
- Consolidate the child/young person's ability to express themselves so they can request an item or activity using language (including AAC). Encourage appealing activities with lots of communication opportunities (see sections titled "Attention" and "Play").
- Able to use language for a range of reasons. Model (implicit learning) using language for lots of reasons using any AAC that supports the young person's communication. Identify situations to teach specific language functions meaningfully within natural routines.

---

Clare's story

Clare was regularly self-harming, hitting her head. Following a discussion, it was agreed to teach her to say "no" so that she had a clear way of refusing an activity or request. Staff and parents worked hard to introduce this, modelling the use of the symbol and sign, providing Clare with the symbol on her own fob, "No," so it was always available wherever she was and supporting her to use this. "No" was always honoured, so she had autonomy in this. Her self-harming decreased. As she felt comfortable with her ability to refuse an activity and withdraw, she became more willing to try activities, and her participation increased.

No

---

The message can be expressed and received through any means:

- Objects of reference.
- Picture/symbol.
- Speech or writing.
- Sign.

For a child/young person at a very early stage of language, the focus will be on developing **vocabulary**: words that can be used across the day/week for a range of purposes. A word expresses a meaning and provides an opportunity for the parent/carer to respond: "first words enable children to not only express themselves but also elicit feedback from communication partners that supports further language development" (Laubscher & Light, 2020).

Many autistic children and young people start using language to make requests using nouns. They may find it more challenging to use people's names and verbs.

> John (Chapter 1) did not recognise his therapist when she was wearing a skirt. A neurodivergent parent recognised her son in a class photo from his shoes.

## Colour-coded picture support (colourful semantics/colourful communication)

Colour-coded picture support is based on Alison Bryan's "Colourful Semantics" (Bryan, 1997). Autistic children and young people are often more secure in their ability to ask for *objects* and have more difficulty with language around *people* and *actions*. Colour-coded picture support helps teach the language of people (proper nouns), actions (verbs), objects (nouns) and beyond. The colours help the youngster understand the different parts of speech, understand (and use) question words and link words to make (longer) sentences.

It uses the visual strength of many autistic youngsters to support developing understanding and use of spoken language and supports understanding of a text.

Colour-coded picture support can help support language flexibly. Colour coding helps the youngster understand the meanings of words (semantics) and to structure their responses. To support this, the individual will need lots of modelling.

> **People games**: some autistic youngsters have particular difficulty getting to know the people in their environment. Photos can be helpful to support this.
>
> - Have a photo board with the photo and name of all the people involved with the child/young person.
> - Use photos of people as a prompt for pupils who need extra support to:
>   - Choose/remind who is having the next turn in a game (who's next?).

- o   Remind them of the order in which the pupils will line up.
- o   Remind the class who is doing the jobs today/this week.
- o   Choose who the youngster is going to take to soft play.
- o   Report back about an event (who did you see?).
- o   Choose with whom they want to play.

Consider the limitations of photos; for example, people change their appearance: different clothes, hair and accessories.

Pronouns are particularly difficult for some children and young people with autism. They may have difficulties with he/she, him/her, etc., as seen in other children with delayed or disordered language. In addition, they may have difficulties with you/me, you/I, us/them, we/they, which could relate to difficulties with the theory of mind. This is often associated with other indicators of lack of perspective-taking, like a young child's reverse waving (showing the rear of hand when waving). Use names rather than pronouns to avoid ambiguity.

Use colour-coded visual support with choices. Initially offer one choice (e.g. person or action depending on focus)

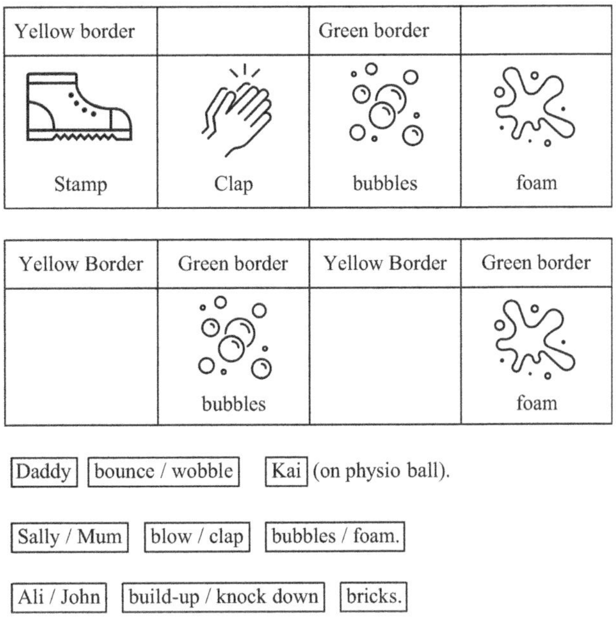

| Yellow border | | Green border | |
|---|---|---|---|
| Stamp | Clap | bubbles | foam |

| Yellow Border | Green border | Yellow Border | Green border |
|---|---|---|---|
| | bubbles | | foam |

Daddy | bounce / wobble | Kai (on physio ball).

Sally / Mum | blow / clap | bubbles / foam.

Ali / John | build-up / knock down | bricks.

**FIGURE 5.11** Colour-coded picture support with choices: clap or stamp?

---

The focus is to introduce a youngster to a range of reasons to communicate: making choices, requesting, commenting, asking and answering questions and giving information. Use motivating activities (e.g. [blowing] bubbles and balloons, [clapping] foam). This could be within a curriculum activity in school or early years and personalised learning opportunities in the educational setting and at home or out and about.

---

Many autistic children and young people with significant language difficulties benefit from visual support alongside spoken language to help reinforce language learning.

- Use symbols (written word on symbol) and consider signing alongside your spoken language.
- Use these motivating activities as choice-making activities. Model the language an individual needs for "Sally squirt water" alongside the pictures/written words. Encourage the individual to repeat this to request and point to each part of the sentence as they say it (e.g. "Mummy blow bubbles").
- Individuals can choose who carries out the activity (e.g. Sally or Mummy blows bubbles? The verb – blow or squirt bubbles? And the object – bubbles or balloons?).
- Encourage the individual to repeat this to request and point to each part of the sentence as they say it.
- Use colour-coded visual support relating to the curriculum (e.g. story or topic). Model using this.
- Look at a page in the story. Provide the youngster with a "who" picture for one (or more) character(s) in the story (e.g. Eric Carle's (1969) Very Hungry Caterpillar). Who can you see?
- Demonstrate how to put the orange pictures on the orange board.
- Provide one or more "what doing" pictures: e.g. eating.
- Model how to put the yellow pictures on the yellow board.
- This will make sentences, e.g. (The) Caterpillar (is) eating.
- Add objects (Caterpillar eating plum).

Action/verb: autistic children and young people often use fewer verbs than nouns. Colour coding helps understand which are the action words; some of them are more dynamic than others!

Select functional verbs (including "help") and practice with repetition to reinforce these.

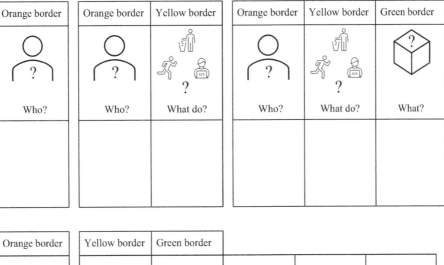

**FIGURE 5.12** Colour-coded picture support: Hungry Caterpillar.

Have colour-coded visual support materials available so the youngster can be supported to make sentences including person and action.

Make an "action book" with photos of the young person doing different actions in their education setting (school/nursery) and at home. Use colour-coded materials to help the youngster make *who* + *what doing* sentences to describe the photos. An adult should support the youngster's sentences daily.

Use *who* and *what doing* questions in class and provide opportunities for the youngster to rehearse answers to increase participation and confidence.

Consider how to include a focus on "who" and "what is happening" across the day/week at home and school/nursery.

Provide a good model of simple sentences – i.e. if a youngster uses one word ("cake"), reflect back two ("cutting cake").

Language can be developed by extending sentences and developing vocabulary.

## Vocabulary

As with any young person, vocabulary development will continue throughout childhood and beyond. Consider a young person's starting point, understanding and use. Consider the context: what helps/hinders a youngster's understanding and use of vocabulary? Be aware of their likely better vocabulary around specialist interests. Use this to scaffold vocabulary development but be careful not to overestimate vocabulary understanding or use based on advanced vocabulary use in one area.

Consider all aspects of vocabulary, not just nouns.

At this early stage, be aware of ambiguity and strive to avoid it! Work with the community on increasing awareness of the complexity of neurotypical language usage.

However symbols are used, consistent modelling to demonstrate use is essential. Therapists and staff should only expect children/young people to start using symbols communicatively once they have had plenty of opportunities to observe their use.

## Joining words

At this stage, a young person links words (including AAC) to express themselves for various purposes.

*Important for all*: being with other people/emotional regulation/joint attention/language for self-advocacy.

Develop the young person's autonomy:

- Ability of the people around them to provide an environment that promotes responsive, social interaction to initiate and sustain social interaction (not just interaction to meet wants/needs).
- Ability of people around them to provide an environment with lots of opportunities to communicate: appealing activities available.
- Ability of child/young person to express themselves so they can request an item or activity using language (including AAC). Encourage appealing activities with lots of communication opportunities (see sections titled "Attention" and "Play").
- Ability to use language for a range of reasons. Model (implicit learning) using language for lots of reasons using any AAC that supports the young person's communication.

Identify situations to teach specific language functions meaningfully within natural routines.

- Ability to use language for narrative: retelling events, moving away from the "here and now" to more abstract (e.g. Blank level 3).
- Ability to use language for reasoning (e.g. Blank level 4).

A systematic literature review of oral narrative interventions found that "icons, visuals, [and] clinician modelling" were used in successful interventions (Favot et al., 2021).

## Ambiguity

Particularly relevant to youngsters with autism is ambiguous language. This may be a fascination for some young people, particularly interested in wordplay and verbal humour. For others, **ambiguity may be a source of immense confusion, frustration and anxiety:**

- Homonyms: bat (e.g. flying mammal/cricket bat) may not be so good at using context to work out a meaning, e.g. "the blind man is here."
- Implied meaning: "wash your hands in the toilet" implied meaning is in the handbasin in the toilets, but a child may misinterpret it.
- Idiom: no literal meaning, but implies the story behind the words: *green fingers, raining cats and dogs, a penny for your thoughts, a frog in your throat.*
- Metaphor: literally describes something that it is not for effect: "she is a ray of sunshine."
- Oxymoron: apparently contradictory words used together for effect: *awfully good, friendly fire, virtual reality.*
- Hyperbole: an exaggeration used for effect: "My mum will kill me when she sees the mess." "I'm so hungry I could eat a horse."
- Irony: a statement that directly contradicts reality: "lovely weather!"
- Stress and tone of voice can change the meaning significantly while the words stay the same. These meanings are subtle to some autistic youngsters and can be hidden communication clues.

    "<u>Give</u> that book to me" (do not throw it).

    "Give <u>that</u> book to me" (not the other book).

    "Give that <u>book</u> to me" (not the cup).

    "Give that book to <u>me</u>" (not to anyone else).

- Sarcasm: irony directed at a person with the intent to criticise: "I'm glad to see you made an effort...."

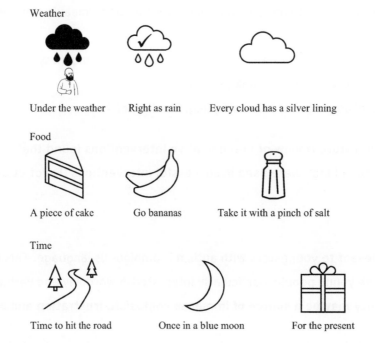

**FIGURE 5.13** Ambiguous language.

## *What to do*

- Ensure that parents/carers/staff are aware of the child/young person's difficulties with understanding language, particularly youngsters with generally good/excellent language skills.
- Adults **must** use language carefully to ensure a young person can access it.
- Ambiguous language can be supported through awareness raising, discussion, highlighting and teaching of meanings as it arises.
- Some phrases can be learned effectively so that the youngster's understanding can improve and awkward misunderstandings are avoided, but it is impossible to anticipate all possible incidents of ambiguity.
- It is therefore essential to ensure that children and young people can identify when they are unsure and have strategies to manage this: "sorry, I don't understand," "what does… mean?"

---

**Reminder:** it is not the young person's fault when they do not understand something that the neurotypical person says that does not make (literal) sense.

---

Consider where the young person is now (rather than comparing to a neurotypical young person).

**TABLE 5.5** Summary of language levels

|  | Develop skills of the communication partner | Impact on skills of child/young person |
|---|---|---|
| Pre-intentional | • Follow the child/young person's lead.<br>  ○ Pause<br>  ○ Observe<br>  ○ Join in (copy with care)<br>Rapport<br>Play | • Initiate interaction.<br>• Develop non-verbal communication skills.<br>• Develop social relationships. |
| Intentional (non-verbal) | • Follow the child/young person's lead.<br>• Provide appealing activities with opportunities to communicate for different reasons.<br>• Model intentional language: e.g. requesting using a range of means.<br>• Consider using clear boxes (symbols attached) with preferred items to teach gestures.<br>Rapport<br>Joint attention<br>Play | • Request using conventional means: eye gaze, reach, touch, give gesture.<br>• Make a choice.<br>• Anticipation. |
| First words | Provide (visual) support (e.g. colour-coded picture support/colourful semantics) to support the development of useful first words and short phrases. Consider core vocabulary: words that can be used for many functions.<br>Model<br>Support understanding<br>Environmental support<br>Rapport<br>Joint attention<br>Play | Using "words" (symbolic means) for a range of reasons. |
| Joining words | Colour-coded visual support develops the young person's ability to use people and action words in phrases and in a narrative.<br>Model<br>Support understanding<br>Environmental support<br>Rapport<br>Joint attention<br>Play | Able to use words (words in the broadest sense: e.g. spoken, signed, symbols) in phrases and beyond, including people and action words.<br>Respond to Blank level<br>3 → 4 → narrative. |

## Useful resources

*Colourful Semantics: A Resource for Developing Children's Spoken and Written Language Skills* (NHS Forth Valley, 2020)

*Language for Thinking* (Parsons & Branagan, 2016)

Black Sheep narrative packs, e.g. *Secondary Talk Narrative* (Shanks, 2010)

Twinkl for Blank levels and colourful semantics (Twinkl, 2022).

## Unclear speech

Autistic children may have unclear speech. As with any child, this may be due to difficulty at any one or more levels:

- Anatomy or sensory (e.g. deafness, hearing impairment, cleft palate) → articulation or phonological disorder.
- Motor: execution difficulties → dysarthria, or planning difficulties, including developmental verbal dyspraxia.
- Perceptual → articulation disorder, phonological disorder.
- Phonetic → articulation disorder.
- Phonemic → phonological disorder (Bowen & Snow, 2017).

It is known that autistic children are at risk of motor difficulties (Zampella et al., 2021), which may involve speech. A limited phonetic repertoire predicts expressive language skills in autistic children with a minimal verbal ability (Saul & Norbury, 2020). The diagnosis of motor speech difficulties is extremely challenging in children and young people with limited expressive language, and it may only be possible to identify suspected motor/planning speech difficulties.

Guidelines for an evidence-based speech assessment of an autistic child (Broome et al., 2017) for clinical and research practice have been developed. The authors acknowledge that this is a challenge within a clinical setting and anticipate that as further evidence is gathered, this will allow the development of best-practice clinical guidelines for the speech assessment of autistic children.

Children or young people at an intentional or pre-intentional (prelinguistic) level of development:

- An assessment of oral motor skills.
- A speech sample of at least 50 speech-like vocalisations.
- Is the child able to imitate phonemes?

For autistic children with speech:

- An assessment of oral motor skills.
- An assessment of connected speech.

- An assessment of single words (100 words), including polysyllabic words.
- Repetition of words to check for consistency of production (Dodd et al., 2009).
- A sentence repetition task.
- A phoneme repetition (stimulability) task.
- Error analysis.
- Intelligibility rating.

This provides

- Phonetic repertoire.
- Syllable shape inventory.
- Stress pattern analysis.

Comparing imitated and spontaneous speech helps when considering the differential diagnosis of a motor speech disorder:

- Better imitation than spontaneous speech is likely to indicate inconsistent speech disorder rather than apraxia/motor planning difficulty.
- Groping, posturing, prolongations and repetitions indicate apraxia/motor planning difficulty rather than inconsistent speech disorder.
- Sequencing errors are likely to indicate a motor planning difficulty; phoneme selection error is likely to indicate an inconsistent speech disorder (Dodd et al., 2009).

The evidence base for interventions for children and young people with autism and motor speech disorders is limited (Beiting & Maas, 2020). A priority for a child with minimal speech is to have the means to express themselves. Beiting and Maas summarise why working on motor speech disorders can be challenging for autistic children, including their difficulties with joint attention and using eye gaze to interpret models of speech and imitation. Where direct speech work is needed, a naturalistic approach reduces interpersonal pressure and increases engagement and generalisation.

There is currently no strong evidence base for non-speech oral motor tasks in treating speech difficulties (e.g. Lee and Gibbon 2015 and Parra-López et al 2022). A core vocabulary approach can be beneficial, particularly when speech production is inconsistent (Dodd et al., 2009).

---

Core vocabulary approach:

- Select 70 words that are **functionally important**.
- (up to) Ten words are selected each session to target for a period; the focus is on the best possible and **consistent** production. The aim is for consistency; it may not be error-free production.
- Practice and model regularly within the naturalistic setting. (Dodd et al., 2009)

---

## Conversation

All individuals have preferences in conversation and social interaction. Many autistic children and young people's priorities may differ from neurotypical peers, so conversation and interaction can look different. For example, a conversation may seem less balanced, with one person maintaining the speaker role for longer, providing information about a particular interest in a sustained monologue (sometimes known as "info dumping"). They may be so focused on content that they miss their conversational partner's non-verbal signals attempting to add to the conversation. It may be that the autistic young person is aware that their knowledge of the topic is far superior to the other person's knowledge. When autistic people talk, conversational turns are generally (much) longer.

Some people prefer conversation that does not require an instant response (e.g. via text, email or social media): asynchronous communication. This allows time to consider the other person's input and plan a reply.

When conversing with neurotypical people, autistic adults reported that knowing the type of conversation, e.g. social chit-chat, help and advice, telling off and problem-solving, enabled them to know what to expect and so to be prepared (Silver & Parsons, 2022).

*What to do*

Before implementing a programme to target conversational or social skills, consider:

- Who is this an issue for?
- What is the purpose of any intervention?

Teaching neurotypical conversational or social skills to autistic children and adolescents contributes to masking and is considered by many autistic adults to be harmful. Instead:

- Promote acceptance of autistic people.
- Develop the skills of people in the community in alerting/agreeing with autistic children and young people of the type of conversation that is starting to support their participation. "Hi Ash, we're here to talk about your work experience at the library. We can think about the job, what work you will do and how we can help you."
- Ensure the youngster is encouraged to express and value their point of view while respecting other people's views **and expecting the same in return.**

## Social understanding

Our role is to support perspective-taking in both directions: double empathy problem (Milton, 2012); ensuring that the responsibility for any issues that arise is not attributed to the autistic individual (who may well have a factually correct, morally sound interpretation of a situation). See Chapter 4.

## Support focus on people

*What to do*

Encourage family/carers to take and talk about photos and videos of people important in their lives. Tagging people and then looking back at the photos (and videos) of the same person in different situations, different clothes, hairstyles, (sun)glasses. Then, randomly looking at photos and talking about the different people:

- What is their name?
- How is the child/young person expected to address the person? What do other people call the person?
- What is their relationship?
- Who are they connected to?

Using a circle of support approach also allows this to be used to support understanding of hidden social rules:

Circle of support: a big poster can be made, and photos of people can be put into the circle.

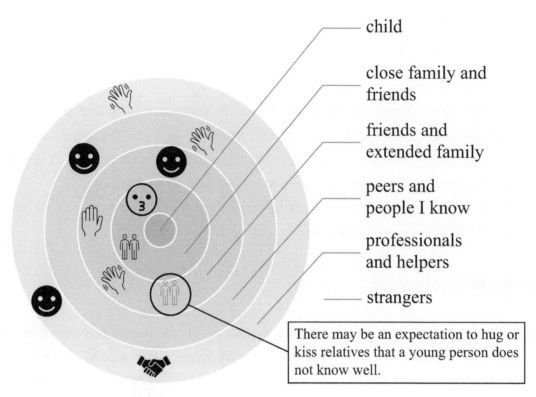

child

close family and friends

friends and extended family

peers and people I know

professionals and helpers

strangers

There may be an expectation to hug or kiss relatives that a young person does not know well.

**FIGURE 5.14** Circle of support.

How to greet different people: hug/high 5/"hello Ms Name" and proximity rules.

This is for safety, and youngsters should not do **more** than this. They may choose to do less (e.g. a young person may not want physical contact, which should be respected).

Supporting understanding of hidden social rules:

1.  Identify who is in each group with the child/young person and plot onto a diagram.
2.  Consider and agree on the unspoken rules.

Perspective-taking can be effectively supported using media (books, YouTube, TV, films, etc.) to explore in a safe, non-personal setting. Provide specific learning using planned and incidental opportunities. Careful use of YouTube (always preview to check the content!) allows the use of content that can be at an appropriate interest level. Use speech and thought bubbles to consider characters' thinking and their words and actions. This allows practice in thinking about other people's points of view.

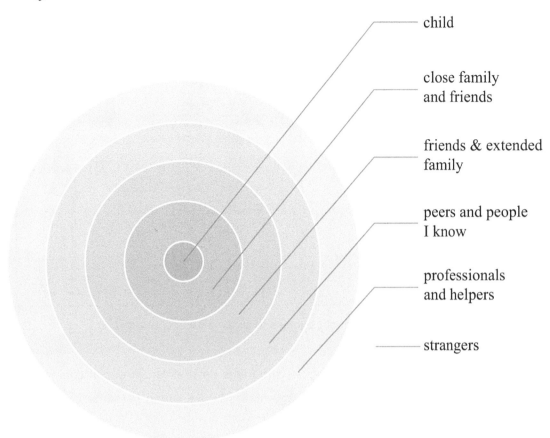

child

close family
and friends

friends & extended
family

peers and people
I know

professionals
and helpers

strangers

| smile | kiss | hug/touch | high 5 | wave | handshake |
|---|---|---|---|---|---|
| smile | kiss | hug/touch | high 5 | wave | handshake |
| smile | kiss | hug/touch | high 5 | wave | handshake |

**Then potentially may work towards developing more flexibility (or not).**

**FIGURE 5.15** Blank circle of support.

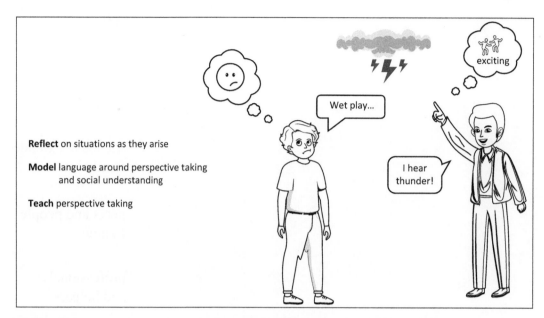

**FIGURE 5.16** Using speech and thought bubbles to support perspective-taking.

Take opportunities to comment on social situations as they arise: social commentary. Model language and thinking and encourage others in the young person's life to do the same.

Increasing social understanding can be helped by being more explicit about the hidden social world and making this more predictable. Supporting understanding helps make life more predictable and increases trust in the world and people.

## Hidden rules

Many social rules are ambiguous.

Consider the hidden rules of touch in day-to-day life. Agree on what is appropriate for the young person in their contexts. For example, shoulders, hands (high 5), elbows, lower arms and upper back may be acceptable.

However, rough-and-tumble play, which often involves whole-body contact, continues into adolescence (and beyond) for some boys.

A sensitively delivered relationships and sex education curriculum is essential, but the young person will need the opportunity to ask questions and discuss to personalise.

Carol Gray's Social Stories™ promote a "safe and meaningful exchange of information" by describing a context, skill, achievement or concept, carefully using specified criteria (Gray, 2022).

> Unconventional strategies such as motor mannerisms, stimming, focus on interests and soothing behaviours are helpful self-regulatory strategies and should not be addressed through interventions. It may be that they are a response to anxiety, in which case it would be appropriate to consider the cause of any anxious or distressed behaviour.

## Comic strip

Use comic strips (e.g. *Comic Strip Conversations* [Gray, 1994]) to jot down what has happened (the good situations and the not so good, but never while the participants are still agitated) and discuss. Use colour-coded (to reflect emotions) speech and thought bubbles to explore what individuals and others said and what they might have been thinking. Validate the young person's perspective rather than "correcting" it. It may be helpful to consider "what ifs…" with possible alternatives to increase social understanding and consideration of the other person's perspective. It can be beneficial for the other person involved to see the young person's perspective, too: double empathy problem. It is helpful to share this with others to see the individual's perspective (in a context where they are learning about the perspective rather than seeking to "correct" it).

*Developing other perspectives*

- Choosing books for different people at the library.
- Choosing ingredients for meals for different people according to their preferences and allergies/tolerances at the supermarket (or planning a shopping list).
- Planning a school trip for class/small group.
- Planning a birthday party.
- Choosing a film suitable for different people to watch, etc. Consider special needs (allergies, intolerances, access needs, age [rating], interests and previous experience).

## Honesty

Neurotypical honesty is very context-bound. It is often surrounded by a complex social agenda, linked to closeness (friendship) and hierarchy and social expectations, and is often not very honest. Autistic honesty is usually very straightforward. Comic strips can be used to investigate this: what each person is thinking and feeling. Some youngsters enjoy role play to explore the impact of different responses on other people, supporting understanding of "hidden" communication.

For example, birthday present game:

In a small group, pretend to have a birthday celebration. Consider an appropriate gift for different people. Choose and "wrap" (party bag) a gift. Present to the recipient. Watch/listen to their reaction. This is an opportunity to practice giving and receiving gifts, predicting what someone might think/feel, reading facial expressions and receiving a gift you do not like! Use speech/thought bubbles and look at the facial expression and body language and listen to voice for clues.

## Outcomes

Specific "SMART" outcomes for children/young people are important, for example, in contributing to an annual review of an Education, Health and Social Care Plan in England. However, some interventions are not focused on SMART outcomes (e.g. intensive intervention), and support may result in positive effects that were not specifically anticipated when targets were set. Consideration of targets so that they have adequate flexibility to ensure depth of understanding and relevance is vital. Penny Lacey (2010) described SCRUFFY targets for pupils working in a special school. The progress towards unspecified outcomes can be documented using the Engagement Model (Standards & Testing Agency, 2020) (see Chapter 4).

## Making the plan

Ensuring that any intervention is incorporated into the child/young person's daily routine is vital.

**TABLE 5.6** SCRUFFY targets

| SMART | | SCRUFFY | |
|---|---|---|---|
| Specific<br>Measurable<br>Achievable<br>Realistic<br>Timely | | Student-led<br>Creative<br>Relevant<br>Unspecified<br>Fun<br>For<br>Youngsters | |

Source: Lacey (2010).

At home:

Support family/carers to plan opportunities to communicate/interact in daily routines, as these may not arise incidentally. Autistic children and young people need opportunities to communicate in various settings with a range of people.

- Encourage carers to notice opportunities for incidental social interaction, e.g. bath time, strapping into car seat/buggy, mealtimes and bedtime. Support the family to develop opportunities for social (non-functional) communication, valuing the interaction for its own sake.

   This can be non-verbal (copying facial expressions), pre-verbal (joining in with "non-sense" conversation) or verbal. This might develop into or from a familiar routine around the activity, encouraging the social/pleasure of the interaction.
- Implement Special Time.
- Build choices into the daily routine: which clothes to wear, which bath toy, milk or water to drink, Weetabix or porridge, what colour/medium to use for writing/drawing/art, scooter or walk. Consider how the young person is making the choices. Consider the family's expectations: giving a young child choice may be unexpected for some families, and an explanation may be needed.
- Plan opportunities to implement/practice communication targets. For example, if a young person is learning to make choices, plan when this can happen across the day: getting dressed, breakfast, music to listen to, hair product/style, etc.
- Support the family/carers to understand and use any communication system the young person has, including modelling using this with the young person. Ensure they have plenty of time to respond.
- Perseverance.

At school:

- Look for opportunities to develop rapport with a range of people. This is likely to need to be planned and supported to be sustained. Pupil needs to develop a relationship with their teacher(s), support staff and several peers (see section titled "Rapport: develop relationships"). More than one secure relationship is vital to maintain confidence should a staff member be absent or on leave.

For example:

- Before school: go in before the bell with a buddy and draw (another preferred task or job for the teacher) for a few minutes.
- Start of day: planned check-in with the teacher; once the relationship is established, stretch to alternative adult: e.g. show drawing, draw together or...

- Lesson: personalised <u>TA</u> support, including planned time for developing rapport. Work towards support from more than one TA.
- Break: climbing frame with <u>peer(s).</u>
- Lesson: supported in class (working more independently).
- Lunch: check in with the lunchtime <u>supervisor.</u>

*What to do*

Having identified targets, these can be plotted onto the youngster's timetable to ensure that they can be implemented and generalised across the day (Table 5.7). For example, George's priority was developing friendships.

With his family and teacher, we identified the first steps:

- Develop George's joint attention.
- Emotional regulation to develop spontaneous participation – further assessment needed.
- Develop the reasons for communication in various settings with different people: adults and peers.

Setting targets for the people in the young person's life is essential as they impact the pupil's day-to-day life.

## Top tips for speech and language therapists supporting an autistic child or young person

- **Relationship:** develop trust. As far as possible, be consistent and reliable. This includes attendance (letting the youngster know when you are coming and what to expect, being on time). What you wear (changing hairstyles, switching between glasses and contact lenses, clothing styles, perfumes/accessories) can make a significant difference. Support others in the child's life to understand the impact of their relationship on the development of trust.
- **Interests:** use the young person's interests to develop relationships. Knowing about a particular interest and using this to help get to know a young person can be a helpful shortcut (e.g. asking about pet, sporting hero, artwork or other interest).
- **Autonomy:** support the young person with the skills to make, communicate and act on their own choices and decisions.

**TABLE 5.7** Integrating targets into daily routine

| | Who supports | Focus | Strategies |
|---|---|---|---|
| Transition into school | Supervised by teacher | Play<br>Peer relationship<br>Rapport | Toys reflecting interests (cars, Lego®, superheroes?). |
| Bell activity – peers completing activity. George and peer have a play tray. | Teacher | | Play alongside another child before peers come in.<br>Model language (peer/teacher): greetings, asking for items, asking for help. Consider visual support.<br>Teacher joins activity, but George leads. Teacher responds to any communication from George (e.g. proximity, glance).<br>First – then board for transition to work. |
| Literacy | TA | Joint attention<br>Ask/answer questions | Activity starter to support joint attention (what's in the bag?).<br>Own copy of book.<br>Positioning.<br>Demonstrate (teacher), model (peers), peer talk (visual support – book).<br>Answer verbally or by pointing in book. |
| Assembly | Independent | | Timer.<br>First – then board.<br>Positioning. |
| Break | Independent | Play<br>Peer relationships<br>Language for a range of reasons! | Climbing frame.<br>Peers modelling.<br>George alongside.<br>Peers supported to be responsive to any bid for interaction from George. |
| Science | TA available | Joint attention<br>Peer relationships<br>Taking turns<br>Language for range of reasons: comment, share interest, report... | Activity starter to capture attention – use interests.<br>Hands-on learning.<br>Demonstration – visual support.<br>Peer modelling.<br>Differentiated questions: Blank levels 1, 2, (3, 4). |
| Lunch | | Language for a range of reasons | Greeting from lunchtime supervisors; any response acknowledged. |
| Break | Independent | Play<br>Peer relationships<br>Language for a range of reasons! | Climbing frame.<br>Peers modelling.<br>George alongside.<br>Peers supported to be responsive to any bid for interaction from George. |
| PE | TA available | Peer relationships<br>Following and giving instructions<br>Taking turns | Visual support to give/follow instructions.<br>Model asking for help.<br>Responsive to any bid for interaction from George. |
| IT | TA | Peer relationships: joint attention | George and partner have own laptops to use, supported to share attention between their activity.<br>Language modelled: Look! Wow! I like.... |

- **Support communication needs and potential breakdown and repair** (no blame). Consider useful phrases: slow down, I'm thinking about that.
- **Support people in the community to learn about autism and autistic people's interaction style**, e.g. monotropism, info-dumping, echolalia.
- **Identify support needs** and share this information effectively.
- **Perspective-taking**: develop perspective-taking skills on all sides.

## Harmful interventions and evidence-based practice

Following diagnosis, parents can search for interventions for their child. This can sometimes result in challenging discussions with the therapist about unfamiliar or worrying interventions, or advice might be asked about interventions. *A Spectrum of Harmful Interventions* (The Westminster Commission on Autism, 2018) is an extremely helpful document highlighting the warning signs of a harmful intervention, guiding principles for picking interventions and reporting suspicious products or therapies.

 ## Useful resources

*Assessment, Diagnosis and Interventions for Autism Spectrum Disorders* (Scottish Intercollegiate Guidelines Network [SIGN], 2016)

*A Spectrum of Harmful Interventions* (The Westminster Commission on Autism, 2018)

*Evidence-Based Pathways to Intervention for Children with Language Disorders* (Ebbels et al., 2019)

*Evidence-Based Practices for Children, Youth, and Young Adults with Autism: Third Generation Review* (Hume et al., 2021)

*Interventions for Children on the Autism Spectrum: A Synthesis of Research Evidence* (Whitehouse et al., 2020)

*Making Sense of Interventions for Children with Developmental Disorders: A Guide for Parents and Professionals* (Bowen & Snow, 2017)

*NICE Autism guidance and quality standards* (National Institute for Health and Care Excellence, 2022)

# References

Alcock, K., Meints, K. & Rowland, C., 2020. *The UK Communicative Development Inventories Words and Gestures*. Havant: J&R Press Ltd.

Aut, N., 2021. *Learning to Play. No. Playing to Learn.* [Online] Available at: https://autistic-village .com/2021/08/12/learning-to-play-no-playing-to-learn/ [Accessed 07 07 2022].

Beiting, M. & Maas, E., 2020. Autism-Centered Therapy for Childhood Apraxia of Speech (ACT4CAS): A Single-Case Experimental Design Study. *American Journal of Speech – Language Pathology (Online), Suppl. Special Issue: Selected Papers From the 2020 Conference on Motor Speech-Clinical Science and Implications*, 30(3S), pp. 1525-1541.

Best, W., Ping Sze, W., Edmundson, A. & Nickels, L., 2019. What Counts as Evidence? Swimming against the Tide: Valuing Both Clinically Informed Experimentally Controlled Case Series and Randomized Controlled Trials in Intervention Research. *Evidence-Based Communication Assessment and Intervention*, 13(3), pp. 107-135.

Blank, M., Rose, S. A. & Berlin, L. J., 1978. *The Language of Learning: The Preschool Years*. Australia: Grune & Stratton.

Bowen, C. & Snow, P., 2017. *Making Sense of Interventions for Children with Developmental Disorders: A Guide for Parents and Professionals*. Guildford: J&R Press ltd.

Broome, K., McCabe, P., Docking, K. & Doble, M., 2017. A Systematic Review of Speech Assessments for Children With Autism Spectrum Disorder: Recommendations for Best Practice. *American Journal of Speech-Language Pathology*, 26, pp. 1011-1029.

Bryan, A., 1997. Colourful Semantics. In: S. Chiat, J. Law & J. Marshall, eds. *Language Disorders in Children and Adults: Psycholinguistic Approaches to Therapy*. London: Whurr, pp. 143-161.

Carle, E., 1969. *The Very Hungry Caterpillar*. London: Puffin.

Carter, A. S. et al., 2011. A Randomized Controlled Trial of Hanen's 'More Than Words' in Toddlers with Early Autism Symptoms. *The Journal of Child Psychology and Psychiatry*, 52(7), pp. 741-752.

Cooper, J., Moodley, M. & Reynell, J., 1978. *Helping Language Development*. London: Hodder Arnold.

Cullen, R., 2021. *The Autistic Communication Hypothesis*. [Online] Available at: https://aucademy.co .uk/rachel-cullen-they-them/ [Accessed 15 08 2022].

Davies, G., 2022. *Gina Davies Autism Centre*. [Online] Available at: https://www.ginadavies.co.uk/ [Accessed 27 10 2022].

Dodd, B., Holm, A., Crosbie, S. & McIntosh, B., 2009. Core Vocabulary Intervention for Inconsistent Speech Disorder. In: A. L. Williams, S. McLeod & R. J. McCauley, eds. *Interventions for Speech Sound Disorders in Children*. Baltimore: Brookes, pp. 117-136.

Ebbels, S. H. et al., 2019. Evidence Based Pathways to Intervention for Children with Language Disorders. *International Journal of Language and Communication Disorders*, 54(1), pp. 3-19.

Elks, L. & McLachlan, H., 2007. *Test of Abstract Language Comprehension*. St. Mabyn: ELKLAN.

Elks, L. & McLachlan, H., 2009. *Language Builders for Verbal ASD*. St. Mabyn: ELKLAN.

Favot, K., Carter, M. & Stephenson, J., 2021. The Effects of Oral Narrative Intervention on the Narratives of Children with Language Disorder: A Systematic Literature Review. *Journal of Developmental and Physical Disabilities*, 33, pp. 489-536.

Garnett, R., Davidson, B. & Eadie, P., 2022. Telepractice Delivery of an Autism Communication Intervention Program to Parent Groups. *Research in Autism Spectrum Disorders*, 91, pp. 1-18.

Gray, C., 1994. *Comic Strip Conversations*. Arlington: Future Horizons.

Gray, C., 2022. *Carol Gray Social Stories*. [Online] Available at: https://carolgraysocialstories.com/ social-stories/ [Accessed 24 10 2022].

Green, J. et al., 2010. Parent-mediated Communication-focused Treatment in Children with Autism (PACT): A Randomised Controlled Trial. *Lancet*, 375, pp. 2152-2160.

Hume, K. et al., 2021. Evidence-Based Practices for Children, Youth, and Young Adults with Autism: Third Generation Review. *Journal of Autism and Developmental Disorders*, 51, pp. 4013-4032.

Jaswala, V. K. & Akhtarb, N., 2019. Being versus Appearing Socially Uninterested: Challenging Assumptions about Social Motivation in Autism. *Behavioral and Brain Sciences*, 42(e82), pp. 1-73.

Kossyvaki, L. & Papoudi, D., 2016. A Review of Play Interventions for Children with Autism at School. *International Journal of Disability, Development and Education*, 63(1), pp. 45-63.

Lacey, P., 2010. Smart and Scruffy Targets. *The SLD Experience*, 57(1), pp. 16-21.

Laubscher, E. & Light, J., 2020. Core Vocabulary Lists for Young Children and Considerations for Early Language Development: A Narrative Review. *Augmentative and Alternative Communication*, 36(1), pp. 43-53.

Lee ASY, Gibbon FE. Non-speech oral motor treatment for children with developmental speech sound disorders. Cochrane Database of Systematic Reviews 2015, Issue 3. Art. No.: CD009383. DOI: 10.1002/14651858.CD009383.pub2.

LeGoff, D. B., Gomez De La Gomez, G., Krauss, G. & Baron-Cohen, S., 2014. *LEGO (R)-Based Therapy: How to Build Social Competence through LEGO (R)-based Clubs for Children with Autism and Related Conditions*. London: Jessica Kingsley Publishers.

McLachlan, H. & Elks, L., 2010. *Test of Abstract Language Comprehension 2*. St. Mabyn: ELKLAN.

Milton, D., 2012. On the Ontological Status of Autism: The 'Double Empathy Problem'. *Disability & Society*, 27(6), pp. 883–887.

Mouriére, A., 2018. Autism and Intensive Interaction & Intensive Interaction with More Able People. In: D. Hewett, ed. *The Intensive Interaction Handbook*. Second Edition ed. London: Sage Publishing.

Mourière, A. & Hewett, D., 2021. Autism, Intensive Interaction and the Development of Nonverbal Communication in a Teenager Diagnosed with PDD-NOS: A Case Study. *Support for Learning*, 36(3), pp. 400–420.

Narzisi, A. et al., 2021. Could You Give Me the Blue Brick? LEGO®-Based Therapy as a Social Development Program for Children with Autism Spectrum Disorder: A Systematic Review. *Brain Sciences*, 11.

National Institute for Health and Care Excellence, 2021. *The NICE Guideline on the Management and Support of Children and Young People on the Autism Spectrum*. London: NICE.

National Institute for Health and Care Excellence, 2022. *Autism*. [Online] Available at: https://www.nice.org.uk/guidance/conditions-and-diseases/mental-health-and-behavioural-conditions/autism [Accessed 25 10 2022].

NHS Forth Valley, 2020. *Colourful Semantics: A Resource for Developing Children's Spoken and Written Language Skills*. Abingdon: Routledge.

Nind, M. & Hewett, D., 2003. *A Practical Guide to Intensive Interaction*. Birmingham: British Institute of Learning Disabilities.

O'Keeffe, C. & McNally, S., 2021. A Systematic Review of PlayBased Interventions Targeting the Social Communication Skills of Children with Autism Spectrum Disorder in Educational Contexts. *Review Journal of Autism and Developmental Disorders*.

Parra-López, P.; Olmos-Soria, M.; Valero-García, A.V. Nonverbal Oro-Motor Exercises: Do They Really Work for Phonoarticulatory Difficulties? Int. J. Environ. Res. Public Health 2022, 19, 5459. https://doi.org/10.3390/ijerph19095459

Parsons, S. & Branagan, A., 2016. *Language for Thinking: A Structured Approach for Young Children*. 2nd ed. Abingdon: Routledge.

Pickles, A. et al., 2016. Parent-mediated Social Communication Therapy for Young Children with Autism (PACT): Long-term Follow-up of a Randomised Controlled Trial. *Lancet*, 388, pp. 2501–2509.

Pyramid Educational Consultants®, n.d. *What is PECS®*. [Online] Available at: https://pecs-unitedkingdom.com/pecs/ [Accessed 29 09 2022].

Rommelse, N. N. J. et al., 2010. Shared Heritability of Attention-deficit/Hyperactivity Disorder and Autism Spectrum Disorder. *European Child and Adolescent Psychiatry*, 19, pp. 281–295.

Saul, J. & Norbury, C., 2020. Does Phonetic Repertoire in Minimally Verbal Autistic Preschoolers Predict the Severity of Later Expressive Language Impairment? *Autism*, 24(5), pp. 1217–1231.

Scottish Intercollegiate Guidelines Network (SIGN), 2016. *Assessment, Diagnosis and Interventions for Autism Spectrum Disorders*. Edinburgh: SIGN.

Shanks, B., 2010. *Secondary Talk Narrative*. [Online] Available at: https://www.blacksheeppress.co.uk/product/secondary-talk-narrative-ks3-4/.

Silver, K. & Parsons, S., 2022. Perspectives of Autistic Adults on the Strategies that Help or Hinder Successful Conversations. *Autism & Developmental Language Impairments*, 7, pp. 1–14.

Standards & Testing Agency, 2020. *The Engagement Model: Guidance for Maintained Schools, Academies (Including Free Schools) and Local Authorities*. [Online] Available at: https://www.gov.uk/government/publications/the-engagement-model [Accessed 19 05 2022].

Sterponi, L. & Shankey, J., 2014. Rethinking Echolalia: Repetition as Interactional Resource in the Communication of a Child with Autism. *Journal of Child Language*, 41(2), pp. 275–304.

Stiegler, L. N., 2015. Examining the Echolalia Literature: Where Do Speech-Language Pathologists Stand?. *American Journal of Speech-Language Pathology*, 24(4), pp. 750–762.

Sussman, F., 2012. *More Than Words®: A Parent's Guide to Building Interaction and Language Skills for Children with Autism Spectrum Disorder or Social Communication Difficulties*. 2nd ed. Toronto: Hanen Centre.

The Westminster Commission on Autism, 2018. *A Spectrum of Harmful Interventions*. London: Westminster Commission on Autism.

Twinkl, 2022. *Blanks Levels*. [Online] Available at: https://www.twinkl.co.uk/search?q=blanks+levels [Accessed 18 10 2022].

Whitehouse, A. et al., 2020. *Interventions for Children on the Autism Spectrum: A Synthesis of Research Evidence*. Brisbane: Autism CRC.

Williams, G. L., Wharton, T. & Jagoe, C., 2021. Mutual (Mis)understanding: Reframing Autistic Pragmatic "Impairments" Using Relevance Theory. *Frontiers in Psychology*, 12.

Zampella, C. J. et al., 2021. Motor Skill Differences in Autism Spectrum Disorder: A Clinically Focused Review. *Current Psychiatry Reports*, 23(64).

# EMOTIONS

DOI: 10.4324/9781003154334-8

**Key points**

- Autistic children and young people may have difficulties understanding and expressing their emotions.
- They may have difficulties interpreting other people's expressions of emotion, but this is not inevitable.
- Other people may have difficulties understanding the emotions expressed by autistic children and young people.
- Emotional regulation may be a difficulty.
- Anxiety is common in autism and is likely to result from living in a world that does not understand neurodivergence.
- Work with the multidisciplinary team to support children and young people with their emotions/emotional regulation.

**Focus on**

- Supporting the people in the young person's environment to understand their perspective, how the youngster expresses emotions and what they need.
- Developing the young person's ability to identify their emotions, what they need and ensuring that these needs are met, including their ability to self-advocate.

# Introduction

Autistic children and young people may have differences in their understanding or expression of emotions. Diagnostic criteria specify that an individual will have difficulties with social-emotional reciprocity, which might include reduced sharing of emotions: DSM-5 (American Psychiatric Association, 2013) and/or responding to the feelings and emotional states of others: ICD-11 (World Health Organization, 2022) .

The impact of these difficulties can affect the individual's interaction with other people. For example, an infant who is unresponsive to a caregiver's smile is likely to interact less with other people, and people are less likely to engage with an infant who does not actively respond. If a child does not express their own emotion using facial expressions, other people may be less responsive to them, it may be more challenging to make and maintain friendships, and relationships may be less secure.

Some autistic children and young people need a great deal of support to deal with their own emotions. Anxiety and depression are highly prevalent among autistic individuals. However, the diagnosis of these mental health difficulties can be complicated by the individual's verbal and non-verbal communication skills, which could be related to their autism or an additional need (diagnostic overshadowing).

The differences experienced are hugely varied. For example:

- Limited range of facial expressions, body language and intonation. For example, others might interpret the child or young person as very serious, bored or robotic.
- Superficially appropriate affect. Another youngster might not have any apparent differences on first meeting, but they could observe the emotional expression around them and match their behaviour to this (masking).
- Inappropriate response to emotions, particularly laughing. This can be interpreted as unkind or challenging behaviour. However, it is often an anxious response to unexpected behaviour from another person, or the young person could be responding to a different aspect of the situation (e.g. seeing the slapstick comedy in someone tripping and spilling something but missing the emotional response of that person).
- Distressed behaviour could be wide-ranging, for example, aggression towards self and others and damage to property, which relates to very high levels of emotion.

There are several possible causes for differences that might occur individually or in combination:

- Difficulties understanding own emotions may be associated with difficulties interpreting internal senses within the body (interoception) and/or with understanding the language of emotions (may need modelling and visual support).
- Difficulty interpreting other people's emotions (may need modelling, visual support and perspective-taking).
- Difficulty expressing own emotions (may need modelling, visual support).
- Difficulty regulating own emotions (needing modelling, visual support + interoception).

---

**Alexithymia**: difficulty identifying and describing a person's own emotions. Alexithymia is reported in 10% of the general population and about 50% of the autistic population (cited in Mul et al., 2018). It is also associated with other diagnoses (e.g. eating disorders and depression). It appears to be associated with sensory differences in some individuals, so they may not experience or recognise signals within the body usually associated with emotions: interoception.

**Interoception**: the physical feelings of what is happening inside the body, e.g. recognition of body temperature, pain, hunger and anxiety. This is a sensory difference (see Chapter 7).

## Understanding other people's emotions

Autistic children and young people frequently **do** understand the emotions of others. They may be highly sensitive to this and extremely empathic. This empathy often contributes to the masking of difficulties as the young person notices and responds to other people's emotions and works hard to respond to this and fit in. This is potentially exhausting and can make the diagnosis more complicated as this can be seen as evidence of social-emotional reciprocity, making professionals less likely to diagnose autism. This can be seen particularly in girls and women.

Supporting the autistic youngster and those around them in managing emotions is a priority.

The way that some youngsters respond to the emotions of others may be unconventional. This can be for a variety of reasons, for example:

- Their facial expression/body language interpretation may differ from that of neurotypical children and young people.
- Their interpretation of a situation may be different:
  - A youngster may laugh as an anxious response when they do not understand.
  - A young person may laugh to cover up confusion about an unfamiliar response (e.g. seeing a loved one crying).
  - A young person may rely on obvious or idiosyncratic information to identify emotions or find it challenging to use language to explain their response to emotions (Figure 6.1).

Autistic adults have described different social and emotional processing: social information is often processed "offline" (i.e. after the event), while neurotypical children and adults will process more social information "online" (as it is happening). As a result, in assessments where the youngster is encouraged to consider a detached social situation (one that they are not involved in), their social and emotional responses may appear to be adequate, good or extremely insightful, despite experiencing social difficulties day to day.

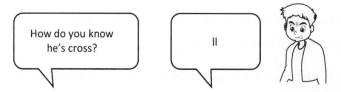

**FIGURE 6.1** Using idiosyncratic information to work out emotions ('II' between eyebrows).

Research supports this, finding that autistic children (in middle childhood) and their parents are aware of their difficulties in pragmatic, language and social behaviours and are more likely than clinicians to identify difficulties. The same study demonstrated that direct assessment often underestimated the difficulties observed, particularly for pragmatic tasks (Sturrock et al., 2020).

> Children and/or young people with relatively good language and cognitive skills are particularly vulnerable to unrealistic expectations from those around them. Their sensory differences, social communication difficulties and/or executive function difficulties can make emotions challenging and can make it extremely difficult to sustain emotional regulation. This can lead to internalised or externalised difficulties. These might be behaviour difficulties very evident to other people, or they may be covert but equally harmful (e.g. very passive, withdrawn, self-harm and/or extreme anxiety).

## What to do

Just as we need to be at the right temperature we all need to be at the "just right" level of alertness/arousal: not too low (e.g. sleepy, bored, unwell) and not too high (e.g. hyper-vigilant, over-active, over-excited, angry, anxious). It is helpful to have a tool to support understanding and communication around alertness. One of these is the thermometer. This visual image can help people understand and identify their energy and/or emotion and that of the children and young people with whom they work.

**TABLE 6.1** Thermometer

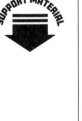
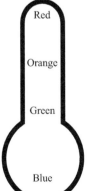

| | |
|---|---|
| **Red** | When extremely unsettled, out of control. |
| | Emotions might include: devastated, terrified, furious, out of control, elated. |
| **Orange** | When agitated, unsettled, but in control. |
| | Emotions might include: anxious, excited, upset, anger, worried, scared. |
| **Green** | The youngster has a good balance of energy and concentration. Just the right amount of sleep, hydration, energy from food, and exercise. Has available support that helps. Regulated, ready to participate. |
| | Emotions might include: happy, OK, calm, good, well, fine. |
| **Blue** | When not alert enough. |
| | Emotions might include: tired, bored, hungry, thirsty, sick/unwell/ill. |

## Step 1: adult's role - notice the needs of all children and young people

The focus is on the adult's role in supporting emotional regulation.

- The adult notices what the child/young person needs to be happy, OK, fine (green).
- Find out: observe and ask (play preferences, Talking Mat, responses to activities, etc.) what the child/young person likes/makes them feel good/happy.
- How do you know when they are happy/well/content/OK/fine? What do you see, hear?

PROACTIVE strategy: as the "green" tools/strategies are identified, sharing these will be prioritised.

Billy is not able to communicate his preferences using conventional means. His class team observed him carefully and listened to his parents to identify some of the things that help him to feel settled in school (Figure 6.2).

**Then notice and document blue and orange levels.**

What do you see when the young person is not so regulated? The child/young person is sharing their emotion, although this may not be in a conventional way.

What does the child/young person need?

Alongside this: adults talk about their levels using the colours, so this is becoming familiar vocabulary. The adult also knows their emotion so that they can add this.

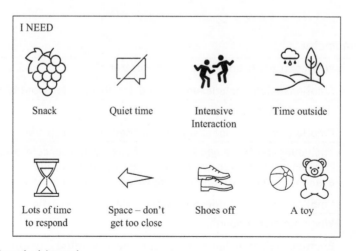

**FIGURE 6.2** Billy: what I need.

**TABLE 6.2** Flow chart of process to support emotions

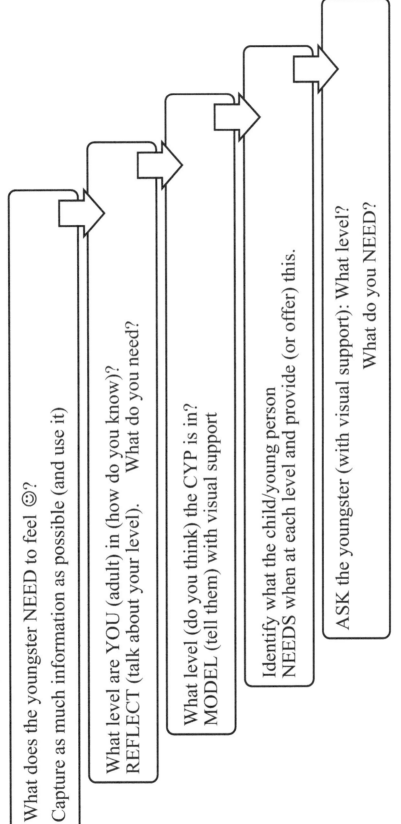

What does the youngster NEED to feel ☺?
Capture as much information as possible (and use it)

What level are YOU (adult) in (how do you know)?
REFLECT (talk about your level).     What do you need?

What level (do you think) the CYP is in?
MODEL (tell them) with visual support

Identify what the child/young person
NEEDS when at each level and provide (or offer) this.

ASK the youngster (with visual support): What level?
What do you NEED?

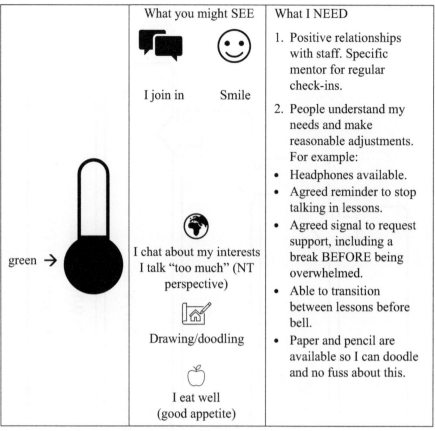

Emily was able to contribute to her thermometer.

**FIGURE 6.3** Emily: what you see, what I need.

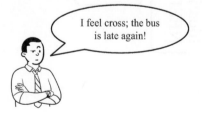

We often need to find out the child/young person's emotion. We can usually identify the level. 🌡

The level (colour) is the first step to identifying how the young person is feeling. The emotional vocabulary is more complex. We reflect on this alongside the levels, talking about our own emotions.

> I feel cross; the bus is late again!

The toolkit will be personal to the individual. Some items are likely to be helpful to many people (e.g. consciously breathing out slowly will help many people: hand breathing), and some may be very specific to an individual (e.g. using a particular acupressure point).

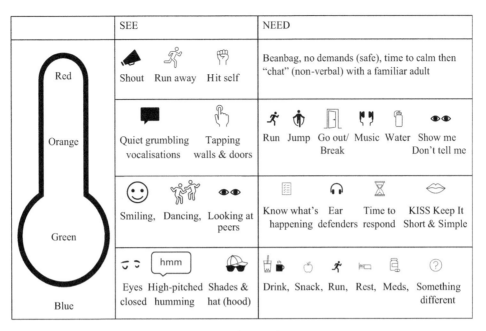

| | SEE | | | NEED | | | | | |
|---|---|---|---|---|---|---|---|---|---|
| Red | Shout | Run away | Hit self | Beanbag, no demands (safe), time to calm then "chat" (non-verbal) with a familiar adult | | | | | |
| Orange | Quiet grumbling vocalisations | Tapping walls & doors | | Run | Jump | Go out/ Break | Music | Water | Show me Don't tell me |
| Green | Smiling, | Dancing, | Looking at peers | Know what's happening | Ear defenders | Time to respond | KISS Keep It Short & Simple | | |
| Blue | Eyes closed | High-pitched humming | Shades & hat (hood) | Drink, | Snack, | Run, | Rest, | Meds, | Something different |

**FIGURE 6.4** Thermometer: what you see, what I need.

---

**Hand breathing**

Trace around the hand with finger of other hand.

Little finger around base of palm to tip of thumb is a breath in (dark grey line).

Tip of thumb all the way around each finger to tip of the little finger is a slow breath out (light grey line).

---

## Thermometer

The use of colours has proved helpful in supporting adults and children/young people to broadly understand their emotions by considering their arousal level and how to respond to it.

## Step 2: model talking about emotions

The next step is for the child/young person to begin recognising their arousal level. This does not require the child/young person to have a sophisticated vocabulary around their emotions (although they might have).

As in Step 1, as far as possible, notice the level of the youngster and MODEL this to them.

• Show thermometer (could be a wall display or your lanyard).

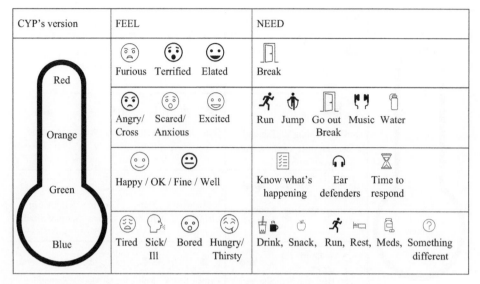

| CYP's version | FEEL | NEED |
|---|---|---|
| Red | Furious  Terrified  Elated | Break |
| Orange | Angry/  Scared/  Excited<br>Cross  Anxious | Run  Jump  Go out  Music  Water<br>Break |
| Green | Happy / OK / Fine / Well | Know what's  Ear  Time to<br>happening  defenders  respond |
| Blue | Tired  Sick/  Bored  Hungry/<br>Ill  Thirsty | Drink,  Snack,  Run,  Rest,  Meds,  Something<br>different |

**FIGURE 6.5** Thermometer: emotion vocabulary available and what I need.

Show the level as you acknowledge their emotion and label it as far as you can tell.

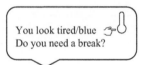

You look tired/blue
Do you need a break?

As far as you can identify, tell the youngster what you think they NEED.

## Step 3: ask - elicit from the child/young person how they are feeling

When they have provided their colour, acknowledge this and comment on what you observe that concurs with this. If appropriate, ask: what do you need (usually offering visual support alongside)?

---

**SUMMARY**

**Reflect:** provide lots of opportunities for autistic children and young people to hear (and see) emotion vocabulary being used appropriately by other people.

All emotions are valid and should be responded to positively.

**Model:** describe what you see in the young person, and tell (and show) them using appropriate emotion vocabulary.

**Ask:** how are you? What do you need?

# Body scan: using interoception to support understanding of emotions

Children and young people can learn to develop an understanding of their own emotions using a body scan, where they are encouraged to notice how their body is feeling (adapted from Goodall, 2019).

Step 1 - awareness of body

Talk about and label basic body parts (for school-aged children and young people link this with the science curriculum). Some children and young people will use more sophisticated language. Use visual support as needed. Initially, work with a peer and draw around each other to produce their own body outline (e.g. on backing paper). Label this.

Basic                                                                 Specialist

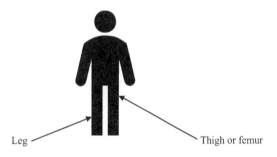

Leg                                          Thigh or femur

If appropriate to the age and developmental level of the youngster, talk about and label the parts that cannot be seen: stomach, heart, lungs and brain. Research these body parts with the youngster to develop their understanding. Use interactive options such as relevant extracts from "Operation Ouch" (CBBC) or science and/or physical education curricula to support understanding.

Step 2

Generate a word (and symbol) bank of vocabulary: body parts (nouns), actions (verbs) and feelings (adjectives/adverbs).

| Basic | Specialist |
|---|---|
| Head - hair - ears (listen) - eyes (see) - nose (smell) - cheeks - mouth (eat, talk, chew, taste, smile, frown, etc.)<br>Chest<br>Tummy<br>Arms - hands - fingers - thumbs<br>Legs - feet - toes | Brain (think, feel) - jaw - forehead - neck (grimace)<br>Lungs (breath) - heart (beats, pumps blood around the body)<br>Stomach, intestines, etc. (digests food)<br>Wrists - elbows - palms<br>Hips - knees - ankles - soles |

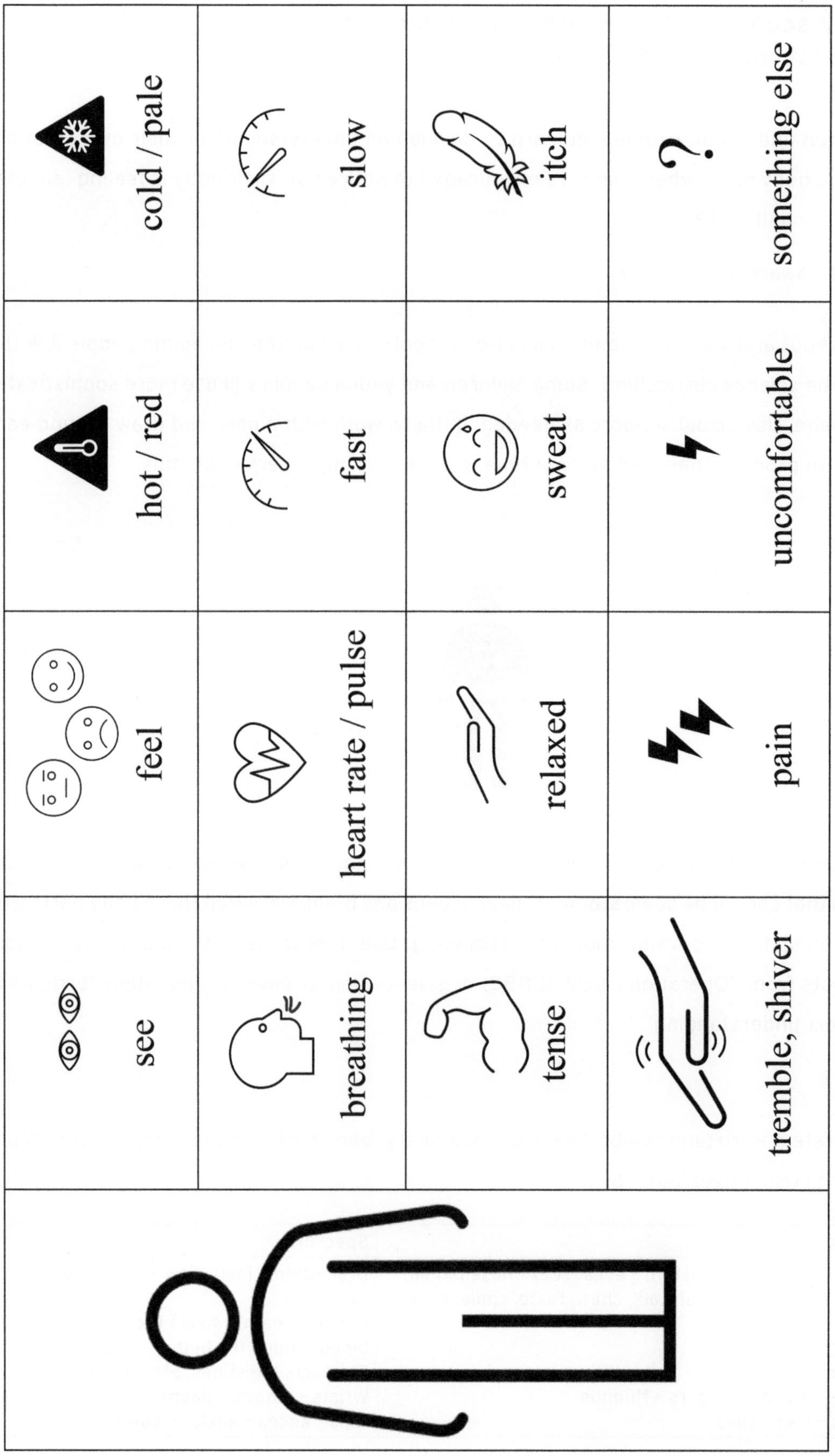

| | see | feel | hot / red | cold / pale |
|---|---|---|---|---|
| | breathing | heart rate / pulse | fast | slow |
| | tense | relaxed | sweat | itch |
| | tremble, shiver | pain | uncomfortable | something else |

FIGURE 6.6 Body scan visual support.

<u>Step 3</u>

Complete your own body scan with the young person. They can watch/listen and comment on their observations of their own body alongside you. As they arise, notice and comment on **your** experiences/sensations associated with your body (e.g. cold hands, rumbling tummy, sweaty face, shivering, goose bumps). What you:

- See: pale, red, sweat, tears, movement, goose bumps, shivering, trembling, etc.
- Hear: breathing, fidgeting.
- Smell: sweat, fragrance.
- Feel: temperature, pain, tense, relaxed, etc.

Link these feelings to the emotion. Use visual support alongside spoken language as needed. For example, the body outline produced previously and a word/symbol bank.

Notice and comment on what **you observe** in the youngster, for example:

- Your forehead looks wet; your cheeks are red; you are breathing fast – you have been running fast. You look tired.

> You look hot; your face is sweaty. Is your heart pumping hard?
>
> I think you are tired. Do you need a drink and a rest?

- Your hood is up, head on table, eyes closed – you could be tired (bored, ill, exhausted, fed up).

Notice and comment on **other people** (as it happens, TV characters, photos, video): eyes droopy, head down, slumped on a chair, hood up – plot on a body scan and find out (ask) or guess how they are feeling.

Elicit information from the child/young person: what do you see, feel, hear and smell?

<u>Photo/video</u>: share photos of familiar people and hunt for clues about the level.

***Step down***: focus on modelling (he looks blue zone: eyes almost closed, lying on a beanbag, head on the pillow). Use visual support.

***Step up***: link to emotions.

| Feeling: | | |
|---|---|---|
| My ears feel… | My head feels… | My eyes feel… |
| My cheeks feel… | | My nose feels… |
| My mouth feels… | 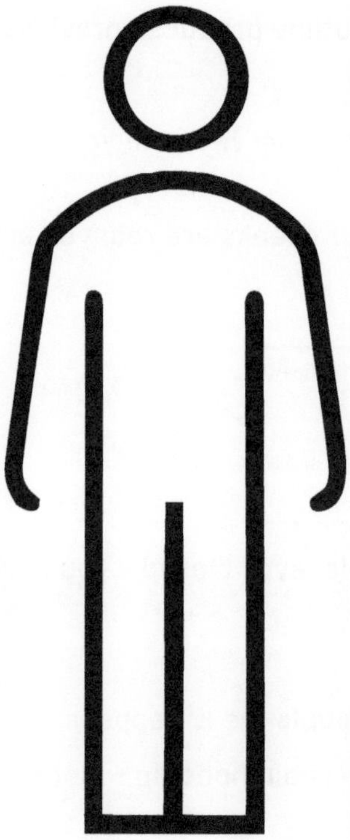 | My throat feels… |
| My neck feels… | | My shoulders feel… |
| My chest feels… | | My arms feel…. |
| My tummy feels… | | My hands feel…. |
| My legs feel… | | My feet feel… |

**FIGURE 6.7** Body map.

**Awareness of feelings → emotions**

Practice a body scan and map this in different situations and experiencing different emotions. Make up a folder with the body map of feelings on one side and a link to needs on the opposite page.

Hungry: brain quiet, tummy rumbling, arms/legs still (low energy, not always the case!).

Excited: brain busy thinking about..., legs fidgety, face smiling, eyes wide open.

Immediately after PE: lungs: breathing fast; heart: beating fast; cheeks: red; forehead: sweaty; etc.

Continue to use visual support to help with communication around feelings and emotions. MODEL using visual support and MODEL talking about feelings and emotions.

## Useful resources

Joint work with colleagues in multidisciplinary team is essential e.g. clinical/educational psychologists, occupational therapists.

*Autism Level Up* (Fede & Laurent, 2020)

*Helping Children Understand and Express Emotions: A Practical Interoception Activity Book* (Goodall, 2019)

*Know Your Normal* (Ambitious About Autism, 2017)

*Zones of Regulation® A Curriculum Designed to Foster Self-Regulation and Emotional Control* (Kuypers, 2011)

*Twinkle: Emotional Regulation* (Twinkl, 2022)

*Supporting Social and Emotional Learning*: ELSA resources (e.g. body sensation resource pack) (ELSA Support, 2022)

# References

Ambitious About Autism, 2017. *Know Your Normal.* [Online] Available at: https://www.ambitiousaboutautism.org.uk/what-we-do/connecting-young-people/youth-led-toolkits/know-your-normal [Accessed 17 05 2018].

American Psychiatric Association, 2013. *Diagnostic And Statistical Manual Of Mental Disorders.* Fifth Edition. Washington: American Psychiatric Association.

ELSA Support, 2022. *Supporting Social and Emotional Learning.* [Online] Available at: https://www.elsa-support.co.uk/ [Accessed 27 10 2022].

Fede, J. & Laurent, A., 2020. *Autism Level Up.* [Online] Available at: https://www.autismlevelup.com.

Goodall, E., 2019. *Helping Children Understand and Express Emotions: A Practical Interoception Activity Book.* Adelaide: Healthy Possibilities.

Kuypers, L. M., 2011. *Zones of Regulation® A Curriculum Designed to Foster Self-Regulation and Emotional Control.* Santa Clara: Socially Thinking Publisher.

Mul, C., Stagg, S. D. & Herbelin, B., 2018. The Feeling of Me Feeling for You: Interoception, Alexithymia and Empathy in Autism. *Journal of Autism and Developmental Disorders*, 48, pp. 2953-2967.

Sturrock, A., Marsden, A., Adams, C. & Freed, J., 2020. Observational and Reported Measures of Language and Pragmatics in Young People with Autism: A Comparison of Respondent Data and Gender Profiles. *Journal of Autism and Developmental Disorders*, 50, pp. 812-830.

Twinkl, 2022. *Twinkle: Emotional Regulation.* [Online] Available at: https://www.twinkl.co.uk/search?q=emotional+regulation [Accessed 26 10 2022].

World Health Organization, 2022. *International Classification of Diseases Eleventh Revision (ICD-11).* 11 Edition. Geneva: World Health Organization.

# SENSORY

DOI: 10.4324/9781003154334-9

**Key points**

• Sensory differences are significant for many autistic children and young people.

• Sensory experiences can be hard to understand, particularly for children with limited language who are not able to describe their needs.

**Focus on**

• Accessing specialist support (e.g. from an occupational therapist [OT]).

• Supporting the young person and their carers to use the strategies and advice.

## Introduction

Five senses have long been known: sight, touch, hearing, smell and taste. Each has an associated organ making the connection between the sense organ and the sense very clear. It is now known that senses are more complex (e.g. proprioception and interoception) and this complexity is particularly evident in many autistic children and young people. The interaction between the senses can make this more complex. This chapter is written from a speech and language therapy perspective. An occupational therapist may have a different perspective and their advice should be sought about a youngster's participation where necessary. Some practitioners, particularly OTs, but others including speech and language therapists (SLTs), can have additional training in sensory processing or sensory integration.

> Many people have sensory-seeking mannerisms, e.g. fiddling with hair, touching the face, biting their nails. This may be because they are a bit (or very) hyposensitive, or experience some sensory difference (tingly, numbness, etc.). Many people have sensory avoidant behaviours: they avoid particular textures, smells, tastes, sights or sounds. They may be hypersensitive to senses, extremely aware of things that might seem inconsequential to other individuals or they may have a mixed pattern of sensory differences.

Autistic children and young people may have more or more persistent sensory seeking or avoidant behaviours. For example:

• Flicking fingers in front of eyes.

• Looking using peripheral vision.

• Walking on tiptoes.

• Stamping feet.

- Removing shoes and socks.
- Fussing about socks.
- Coat on, zipped up, hood up, whatever the weather.
- Shoulders shrugged up to one or both ears.
- Fingers plugged into ears with or without outer ears folded over the ear hole to add an extra layer of sound insulation.
- Eating non-food items (pica).
- Chewing on clothing.
- Responding to a greeting by sniffing a person (body and/or hair).
- Jumping.
- Ripping clothing.
- Rocking.
- Flapping hands.

---

These behaviours could be used as they are:

- Enjoyable.
- Block out unpleasant sensory information in the environment.
- Help gain sensory information from the environment.
- Help with emotional regulation (soothing, alerting, etc.).

---

Sometimes these behaviours may be harmful to the individual or to other people (e.g. head banging, scratching, pinching). If so, then it is important to work with the team (family, carers/staff and other professionals) to work out the functions of the behaviour.

|  | Sensory seeking | Sensory avoiding |
|---|---|---|
|  | Hyposensitive | Hypersensitive |
|  | Generally under-react and seek out more. May seem loud and bold. | Generally over-react and avoid. May seem timid. |
| Proprioception | Behaviour may seem boisterous. Bumps into people and things. Loves to climb and jump and enjoys rough play. Bangs feet down when walking. | Wary of playground equipment (swings, see-saws, etc.). Cautious of busy places. |
| Auditory | Noise-making in an acoustically pleasing space (tunnel, hall, etc.). | Fingers in ears. "Shrug" posture with one shoulder to ear to free up one hand. Making a noise (vocalising means sounds are attenuated, using the acoustic reflex). |

| Visual | Pressing fingers into eyes, exploring the visual patterns (although this could also be a social avoidance). Watching light through blinds, watching dust mites in sunlight, etc. | Hood up, wearing glasses/tinted glasses, hat with a brim. |
|---|---|---|
| Taste | Preference for highly flavoured or spicy food, hot food. | Preference for bland food (often fairly beige). Able to detect a change in flavour (e.g. a different brand, change in recipe, hidden ingredient). |
| Smell | Greeting people by sniffing hair and/or body. | May have a restricted diet based on smell, intolerant of anything outside a limited, familiar range. |
| Touch | Twiddling labels/seam. Chewing on clothing. Seeking out items. Touching things, not aware of personal space. | Must wear "comfy" clothes. Shoes can be difficult. Socks may be tough and have to be put on with such care, seams perfect, can take a long time. |

Liam was an autistic four-year-old who had just started in his mainstream school. His mother had carefully removed all the labels in his clothing as he was so distracted by twiddling them. Unfortunately, as he had no labels available, Liam started putting his hands into the clothing of anyone sitting near him to find a label to twiddle while sitting on the carpet at school. This was extremely disruptive and was resulting in rapidly deteriorating relationships with his peers. It was quickly agreed that it was better for him to have his own twiddle made of clothing labels to hold! While his hands were busy, Liam was able to participate in carpet sessions with some additional adult support and his damaged reputation was quickly restored.

## Interoception

Interoception is the awareness of the internal body state: hunger, thirst, butterflies → anxiety, etc. Some young people with autism have difficulties with this. As a result, they have much less awareness of their own needs. This seems to have an impact on many aspects of independence, for example, they may be slower to recognise when they need to use the toilet; on their appetite regulation: knowing when to eat/drink and/or when to stop. Some youngsters have difficulties gaining weight, others have a tendency to eat too much as they do not appear to have or recognise signals from their body that they have eaten enough.

## Restricted eating (picky eating vs paediatric feeding disorder)

Speech and language therapists working with autistic children and young people are likely to see children with very restricted eating. As with any youngster with concern about their eating (and drinking), this should be considered in terms of dysphagia and a therapist with the skills and experience in assessing dysphagia in children and young people must see them if there are concerns including chest infections, weight loss, coughing or change of breathing when eating/drinking.

A differential diagnosis of picky eating or a paediatric feeding disorder is likely to involve a multidisciplinary approach (Toomey, 2020) to ensure that the child/young person does not have any identified nutritional deficiencies (e.g. paediatrician) and is getting adequate calories and nutrition (dietician). Where their intake is extremely restricted, it may be appropriate to support the child to work towards increasing the range of foods that they are able to eat. Highly specialist SLTs can support with eating (e.g. using SOS Approach to Feeding, 2022).

> One eight-year-old I met appeared to flourish on a diet of formula milk (drunk from a bottle), grated cheese, cheesy puff crisps and nibbling chips from a specific fast-food restaurant.

The child/young person usually has a few (sometimes very few) "safe" foods that they reliably eat. Always **keep the "safe" food safe**. Never mess with it. Never try and hide something in it, disguise a vegetable, medicine or supplement. Accept that the child's safe foods might change (that is, your child might switch their preferences). Also, the manufacturer might change their packaging (gulp!) or worse, their recipe.

But do encourage families to continue to provide very small quantities of another food on a separate dish in front of the child and encourage them with this. Encourage them to speak positively about other foods and the possibility that one day they will find another food that they will try and enjoy however unlikely this might seem!

The stages (e.g. tolerating looking at a food, having it on a dish within their reach, touching it with cutlery, touching it with hands, touching with lips, sniffing it, licking it, putting a piece briefly in mouth etc) to accepting a new food are extremely small, must not be rushed, and each one should be acknowledged and (quietly) celebrated. Neurotypical children are said to take up to 20 tries to accept a new food. Autistic children may take many times this.

Consider foods that have a general similarity to the foods that the child/young person does eat (colour, texture, taste, etc.), but different enough not to appear to be duplicating unsuccessfully a tolerated food, which might put them off this.

We all have foods that we like, those that we tolerate and some that we find nauseating. Repeated exposure to the latter is unlikely to increase our tolerance (and is likely to decrease your appetite), so great care is needed

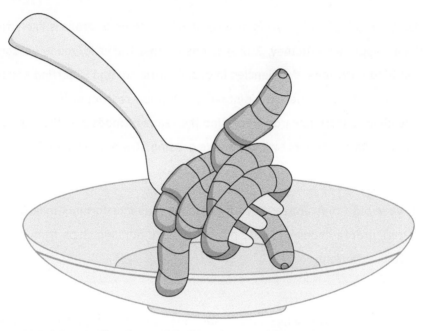

FIGURE 7.1  "I will not ever NEVER eat a"... (Child, 2007)

Andre had a very limited diet but aged ten he was able to respond to a scientific approach to his nutrition. He understood that his body needed a range of different types of food, and so he tolerated eating foods that he knew helped keep him healthy and growing, choosing those that were least intolerable.

## Toileting

A health visitor or school nurse is well placed to advise about toileting. Some areas will have specialist nurses who can provide expert support with toileting. Menstruation is a challenge once girls reach puberty. The sensory aspects of this can be difficult. Considering sensory needs (e.g. period pants may be preferable to pads) and clear explanations to support understanding can be extremely supportive (e.g. see *The Autism-Friendly Guide to Periods* [Steward, 2019]).

## Supporting sensory differences

The environmental supports described previously are all relevant to support youngsters with their sensory differences. However, there are some more specific issues that may need to be taken into account.

Many youngsters can be supported to identify and manage their sensory needs. This may need some scaffolding, particularly at the early stages.

Having control is important for anyone and communication is helpful for everyone. Being able to express preferences is important and expressing sensory preferences is particularly powerful in helping youngsters control their environment.

Some children and young people will know and be able to express what they need.

Many children and young people have strategies that they use to regulate and often these are not harmful, disruptive or problematic. They may be different to others but should be seen as a reasonable adjustment. The Equality Act (2010) does not require that everyone is treated the same, but that reasonable adjustments are made where someone is at a substantial disadvantage as a result of their disability.

Everyone has personal sensory preferences. A liking for the smell of freshly ground coffee (but a dislike of the taste, easily avoided). A loathing of the smell of a shop selling freshly made soaps (but enjoyment of the smell in the shower). A hatred of the thought of the sound of fingernails on a blackboard (a sound not heard for decades). The same emotions can be stirred in autistic children and young people in response to their triggers, but these may be numerous, more extreme and triggered very regularly. Each trigger makes the youngster more susceptible to the next sensory trigger or other triggers. The opportunity to manage this proactively is vital.

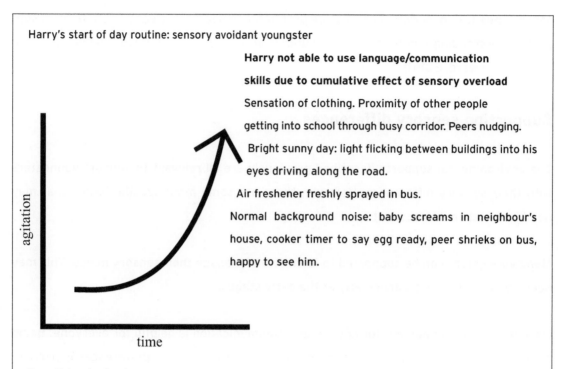

Harry's start of day routine: sensory avoidant youngster

**Harry not able to use language/communication skills due to cumulative effect of sensory overload**

Sensation of clothing. Proximity of other people getting into school through busy corridor. Peers nudging.

Bright sunny day: light flicking between buildings into his eyes driving along the road.

Air freshener freshly sprayed in bus.

Normal background noise: baby screams in neighbour's house, cooker timer to say egg ready, peer shrieks on bus, happy to see him.

Possible strategies:

- Ear defenders and sunshades on bus (or change seating).
- Avoid air freshener.
- Change start of day routine to avoid busy corridor: enter early or late, or use a different entrance.
- Consider clothing: appropriate size (has pupil grown?), reasonable adjustment needed to uniform?
- **Gentle transition into school day: quiet, low arousal, following young person's lead to establish when they are ready for interaction and the demands of school life.**

Encouraging the youngster to fulfil their needs and to do what motivates them: meeting their wants and needs is likely to result in increased participation and so get the best outcomes for the youngster.

Consider and allow sensory preferences as far as possible. Encourage the provision of twiddles, chews, blankets, cushions, sensory cushions, ear defenders etc. The young person will concentrate better while meeting sensory needs than if encouraged to do "good sitting" and sit with feet and hands still, looking at the speaker. Whole body listening is not realistic, achievable or autism-friendly.

Support the youngster to communicate their preferences using any/all available means (e.g. communication passport). Support other people in the environment to be aware of neurodiversity and associated needs.

## Auditory processing

A child or young person with autism may process sounds differently. This may be due to:

- Any current or previous hearing impairment (e.g. glue ear).
- Auditory sensitivity (e.g. hyperacusis). Between 18% and 69% of autistic participants had hyperacusis in studies reviewed by Danesh et al. (2021).
- Social communication difficulties associated with autism also have an impact on auditory processing, so some children may not process sound unless it has been explicitly directed at them or has a particular meaning for them (rustle of a crisp packet!).

Some young people find it extremely difficult to identify what information they need to focus on and so can be extremely distracted by background noise and, in particular, background speech (focus on detail). Therefore, it is helpful to consider turning off the TV, radio, smart speakers and so on.

Using the child's name at the start of an interaction to get their attention is helpful. This can take a significant amount of effort to learn as it can be typical to put the name at the end of an utterance.

Encouraging families to use Special Time can be a straightforward starting point for support. Ensuring that parents speak with their child in their home language is beneficial to supporting the relationship.

Encourage the family to:

- Turn off background noise (radio/TV/smart speakers, etc.).
- Move to within a normal conversational distance to start an interaction.
- Use young person's name at the start of an interaction and face towards the youngster (do not insist on eye contact from the young person).
- Keep it short and simple.
- Say what you mean (avoid non-literal/ambiguous language).
- Give plenty of time to process language.
- Show, don't just tell (put on your shoes – show shoes, use camera/video to support learning of a harder sequence: tying laces).
- Ensure the family use their home language.

Autistic children and young people can have hearing, processing and/or language difficulties in addition to their autism diagnosis.

## Summary

- Sensory differences have a significant impact on autistic children and young people.
- Understanding their sensory needs helps understand the young person.
- An occupational therapist is an important part of the team.

## Useful resources

*Autism Level Up, Regulator for the Classroom* (Fede & Laurent, 2020)

*Eating – A Guide for All Audiences* (National Autistic Society, 2020)

*Picky Eater vs PFD vs AFRID: Differential Diagnosis Decision Tree* (Toomey, 2020)

*Why We Don't Use the ARFID Diagnosis* (Toomey, 2021)

*The Autism-Friendly Guide to Periods* (Steward, 2019)

*Ready to Learn Interoception Kit* (Goodall, 2019)

*Hyperacusis in Autism Spectrum Disorders* (Danesh et al., 2021)

## References

Child, L., 2007. *I Will Not Ever Never Eat a Tomato*. London: Orchard Books.
Danesh, A. A. et al., 2021. Hyperacusis in Autism Spectrum Disorders. *Audiology Research*, 11(4), pp. 547–556.
Equality Act 2010. [Online] Available at: http://www.legislation.gov.uk/ukpga/2010/15/contents
Fede, J. & Laurent, A., 2020. *Autism Level Up*. [Online] Available at: https://www.autismlevelup.com
Goodall, E., 2019. *Ready to Learn Interoception Kit*. [Online] Available at: https://www.education.sa .gov.au/sites/default/files/ready-to-learn-interoception-kit.pdf [Accessed 26 10 2022].
National Autistic Society, 2020. *Eating – A Guide for all Audiences*. [Online] Available at: https:// www.autism.org.uk/advice-and-guidance/topics/behaviour/eating/all-audiences [Accessed 26 10 2022].
SOS Approach to Feeding, 2022. *SOS Approach to Feeding*. [Online] Available at: https://sosappr oachtofeeding.com/ [Accessed 26 10 2022].
Steward, R., 2019. *The Autism-Friendly Guide to Periods*. London: Jessica Kingsley Publishers.
Toomey, K. A., 2020. *Picky Eater vs PFD vs AFRID: Differential Diagnosis Decision Tree*. [Online] Available at: https://sosapproachtofeeding.com/wp-content/uploads/2021/10/11x17-PICKY -EATER-vs-PFD-vs-ARFID-Differential-Diagnosis-Decision-Tree-2021.pdf [Accessed 26 10 2022].
Toomey, K. A., 2021. *Why We Don't Use the ARFID Diagnosis*. [Online] Available at: https://sos approachtofeeding.com/wp-content/uploads/2021/10/Why-We-Dont-Use-the-ARFID-Diagnosis -Article-2021.pdf [Accessed 26 10 2022].

# 8

# MENTAL HEALTH

DOI: 10.4324/9781003154334-10

**Key points**

- Everyone strives for mental health; anxiety is a normal reaction which can be managed within mental health. However, anxiety is problematic for many autistic children and young people when frequent, persistent and/or intense, interfering in day-to-day life.

- Autistic children and young people are particularly vulnerable to life events (adverse childhood experiences) that may lead to trauma, with potentially damaging consequences for mental health.

- It is likely that someone with autism also has another diagnosis. These diagnoses may be overlooked when autism explains difficulties rather than looking at alternative possibilities/diagnoses (diagnostic overshadowing).

- Their autism may make them less resilient as they may have fewer social strategies to support them with these life events.

**Focus on**

- Building positive relationships.

- Developing autonomy through communication skills: joint attention, ability to make choices and express preferences (positive and negative).

- Developing emotional regulation: through environmental support and building the skills of the individual.

- Referring to mental health services for specialist support as needed.

# Anxiety

Some fear or anxiety is a normal response to things that happen and can help respond to situations. For example, the fear of seeing a car approaching too fast makes us produce adrenaline, increasing our heart rate and breathing so that we can respond quickly and effectively and move out of the way quickly.

High anxiety is widespread in many autistic children, young people and adults. Cortisol (stress hormone) studies show that many autistic people "exhibit marked stress responses in otherwise benign, novel and social situations. The hyper-responsivity may contribute to increased anxiety, neophobia or even chronic stress" (Taylor & Corbett, 2014). Neophobia is an excessive fear about anything new or unfamiliar.

About 40% of autistic young people have at least one anxiety disorder (e.g. a specific phobia, obsessive compulsive disorder [OCD] or social anxiety disorder) (van Steensel et al., 2011). These are separate from the individual's autism. However, the autism diagnosis may make it less likely that the anxiety is identified and support provided, as signs of anxiety may be attributed to autism (diagnostic overshadowing).

Anxiety in autism could be caused by factors relating to autism, for example:

- Social communication differences. This can include:
  - extremely high awareness of differences and great effort to camouflage/mask these in order to fit in,
  - the desire for more/better social relationships and/or
  - difficulties with social understanding.
- Difficulty with ambiguity/uncertainty.
- Sensory processing differences that make some sensory experiences very difficult. For some individuals, this leads to distress (e.g. noise sensitivity); for others, it makes it more challenging to make sense of the world (e.g. difficulty interpreting internal body sensations).

The core features of autism can impact a person's trust or certainty. For many autistic people some of their anxiety appears to be related to uncertainty. Prizant describes the uncertainty:

- Trusting the person's own **body**, often as a result of sensory differences.
- Trusting the **world**, which is unreliable (e.g. batteries run out, roads get closed).
- Trusting **people** who are unpredictable and inconsistent. (Prizant, 2019)

Dealing with uncertainty is challenging for many autistic young people, contributing to mental health difficulties without adequate support.

Social media can undoubtedly be a source of support for many autistic people. However, there is increasing evidence that some vulnerable youngsters have unhelpful sources of "support" that can be harmful and increase vulnerabilities.

Anxiety is an almost universal aspect of life for autistic children and young people. Many can find strategies to make this more manageable, with support from people in their lives. The strategies are often those that make life more predictable.

**Camouflaging or masking** autistic behaviours is used consciously or unconsciously by many autistic people in order to fit into a neurotypical world. This might be:

- Learning specific skills (e.g. learning and following socially conventional rules of eye contact).

- Suppressing behaviour(s) (e.g. stimming).
- For some autistic people it could involve a high level of research (e.g. investigating, learning, rehearsing and implementing behaviour changes to navigate social situations).

Masking often begins as an unconscious response to social trauma (Belcher, 2022). There may be potential benefits to this: able to get and sustain employment and/or relationships in a neurotypical society. However, the cost to the individual's mental health is high and may be profound. Autistic adults report the difficult decisions they make to participate in a neurotypical world, resulting in considerable cost to their energy and mental health. For example, the need for quiet time and space away from all demands (despite being able to be an active social participant in work, education and/or leisure opportunities).

Masking "stops us developing our true identities. The pressure to fit in means we rarely have time or energy to do the things we want to do, or to behave like our true selves" (Belcher, 2022).

A co-produced research study between a group of autistic young people from Ambitious about Autism and the academic researchers from the Centre for Research in Autism and Education found that about 80% of the young adults (16-25 year olds) had experienced mental health problems. "Many young autistic people felt that their mental health problems resulted from the pressure to act 'normal' in a neurotypical world" (Crane et al., 2019).

**Adverse Childhood Experiences** are stressful events or situations that occur during childhood and may result in trauma (Brennan et al., 2019).

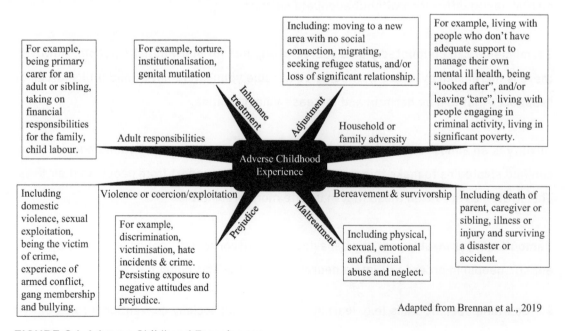

FIGURE 8.1 Adverse Childhood Experiences.

Many children and young people experience adversity, which might lead to trauma. This has potential consequences for mental health. Autistic children and young people are more likely to report one or more adverse experiences. For some youngsters, intrinsic/personal factors (e.g. sensory differences or their awareness of their social communication differences and efforts masking) or extrinsic/societal factors (e.g. negative social experiences, difficulty making/sustaining relationships, bullying, prejudice, difficulty finding/sustaining an appropriate educational placement) relating to their autism contribute to the adversity (Berg et al., 2016).

Children and young people respond to trauma in different ways. For some, it will negatively impact how they see the world so that everything is seen with the experience in mind after the event. For example, after experiencing bullying, a youngster may respond to all social advances from peers as threatening, leading to social withdrawal. This is extremely challenging for a young person with autism with additional communication needs and detrimental to participation and future wellbeing.

> The behavioural response to trauma for autistic children and young people could include increased stimming or other repetitive behaviour, aggression and decreased (social) attention. These may appear to observers to be typical autistic behaviours. Particularly for youngsters with significant communication needs, the opportunity may be missed to identify and support the distress caused by trauma.

A team approach is needed to support the child/young person to consider their whole life, seeking support from other services.

## What to do

*Develop positive relationships*

- Ensure that significant people in the individual's life spend time to develop positive, trusting relationships with the youngster (see Chapter 5).

*Provide control and/or certainty*

- Ensure that the youngster has autonomy in their life as far as possible. Enable them to do the things they love.
- Use support (e.g. visual support) to increase certainty/make life more predictable.

*Support communication*

Listen to the child/young person. Use strategies to support the youngster, for example:

- Visual support (e.g. colour-coded picture support/colourful semantics).
- Talking Mats.
- Mind maps.
- Comic Strip Conversation.

Continue to support the child/young person to express themselves and develop their skills and the skills of those around them.

*Support mutual social understanding and make unspoken rules/information explicit*

- Uncertainty underlies anxiety for many children and young people. Supporting understanding, usually by making unspoken/written information explicit using visual support, positively impacts anxiety (see Chapter 5).
- Using a story can be extremely helpful in developing social understanding.

  Use the story to explain the situation from the pupil's perspective. Use positive language. Tell the child what is happening/what to do/try, not what not to do. Answer the wh-questions about the situation.

  Social Stories® (Gray, 2022) and *Comic Strip Conversations* (Gray, 1994) are extremely helpful (https://carolgraysocialstories.com/carols-club/).

*Support emotional regulation (see Chapter 6)*

## Allow stimming

Stimming is often self-regulating behaviour. Typically, it increases when a child or young person is a bit dysregulated, e.g. anxious, agitated, bored or excited. Provide appropriate support for the emotion, often by supporting understanding the social situation or the routine: what is happening. Allow stimming and find equipment that supports safe and effective stimming, e.g. explore seating for children who like to rock, sensory cushions, provide access to safe "twiddles" as needed. This is preferable to the youngster finding items that may be less safe/desirable. Where stimming becomes self-injurious or dangerous behaviour more proactive intervention is needed, as with any distressed behaviour. Seeking advice from the multi-disciplinary team, psychologist could be extremely helpful in clarifying needs.

# Distressed behaviour and meltdowns

Work with the team around the child/young person and their family to observe, listen and understand what lies behind the behaviours. Like the iceberg, only a small portion is visible. Be sensitive to the broader context of the youngster's family and life. Avoid jumping to conclusions or offering solutions. This requires a team approach and a careful analysis by skilled staff.

What is the function or outcome of the distressed behaviour?

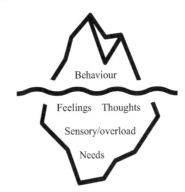

- **Sensory:** provides a preferred sensory experience, blocks a disliked sensory experience, feels good, may be more likely when alone, bored or anxious.
- **Escape:** escapes from activity or interaction, e.g. if too hard, easy, bored, scared.
- **Attention:** gets attention/interaction.
- **Tangibles:** gets access to item or activity.

"The NEST approach" to supporting young people with meltdowns is written by autistic adults in partnership with autistic young people based on collaborative, proactive and low-arousal approaches. It describes what is needed to support an autistic young person who is in a meltdown (Smith et al., 2022).

## Consider unstructured time

Ensure that all children and young people have opportunities to engage with others and access time and space away from social (and other) demands.

Explore alternative options during break times. Unstructured social times can be highly demanding and cannot be considered leisure or a break for some young people. Using these times to support the development of "social skills" should be considered carefully, and the young person should be consulted. There must be consideration of the needs of the young person for time with very low social demands and consideration of sensory needs (they may need a break in a quiet, visually calm place). Individuals have different needs. Some may prefer to be alone; others may like to be in company but not expected to interact, to have a predictable interaction and then be alone, or to participate in a very predictable activity (e.g. a board game at an appropriate level or an activity based around their interest).

| ☺ | 😐 | ☹ |
|---|---|---|
| I like it | OK | I don't like it |

> School break time

Playing games (e.g. football) · Playground · Noise · Lining up

Being with children · Running/exercise · Drink/snack · ⬜

**FIGURE 8.2** Example of a Talking Mat.

It is vital to get the individual's views on the type of break that they need during the school day. Using Talking Mats (see p 61) is an effective way to get a pupil's views:

Ask: How do you feel about… (ask about things within the young person's experience)?

Labels can be clarified and annotated (e.g. playground: climbing frame) and other ideas added (e.g. "wet play"). It may be more appropriate to use symbols. Listen to the young person as they respond to the cards. The discussion may be more important than the resulting mat.

When this is complete check it. So you like…, these… are OK and you don't like….

Then ask: what would you like to change?

Depending on the child/young person's needs, support will be needed to develop a plan. This is likely to require input from the young person and potentially from supportive peers, and observation and input from school staff and parents.

Keep in mind: does the young person want/need break time to be a social or a quiet time?

This can be used to elicit both their opinion and their support needs.

## Mentoring

Having a supportive relationship with (at least one) adult in school is essential and protective of mental health. Having a regular time to build the relationship and to check in/debrief whether or not there are any issues to discuss will help avoid issues building up. Use the 3Cs approach: see what the youngster is interested in, copy (join in) and celebrate (quietly enjoy the experience together). Ensure that the adult is open-minded and prepared to learn about the young person's world and interests.

## Summary

Mental health is a priority for all children and young people. Autistic youngsters are particularly vulnerable to mental ill health, and there must be proactive support in place to improve wellbeing and responsive people including access to specialist mental health services to support when challenges arise.

- Developing autonomy.
- Developing relationships.
- Having opportunities to follow their interests and to be themselves.

 ## Useful resources

*The Anxiety Workbook for Supporting Teens Who Learn Differently: A Framework and Activities to Build Structural, Sensory and Social Certainty* (Ward & Galpin, 2021)

Understanding Autism and Anxiety (Spectrum Gaming, 2022 b)

*Exploring Depression, and Beating the Blues: A CBT Self-Help Guide to Understanding and Coping with Depression in Asperger's Syndrome* (Attwood & Garnett, 2016)

*Autism and Trauma: A Neurodiversity Affirming Guide for Parents+Professionals* (Spectrum Gaming, 2021)

*The NEST Approach: Supporting autistic young people with meltdowns* (Smith et al., 2022)

*Childhood Trauma, the Brain and the Social World* (McCrory, n.d.)

*Keeping Children Safe Online* (NSPCC, 2022)

*Safeguarding young people on the autism spectrum* (National Autistic Society, 2020)

## References

Attwood, T. & Garnett, M., 2016. *Exploring Depression, and Beating the Blues: A CBT Self-Help Guide to Understanding and Coping with Depression in Asperger's Syndrome*. London: Jessica Kingsley Publishers.

Belcher, H., 2022. *Autistic People and Masking*. [Online] Available at: https://www.autism.org.uk/advice-and-guidance/professional-practice/autistic-masking

Berg, K. L. et al., 2016. Disparities in Adversity among Children with Autism Spectrum Disorder: A Population Based Study. *Developmental Medicine & Child Neurology*, 58, pp. 1124–1131.

Brennan, R., Bush, M. & Trickey, D., 2019. *Adversity and Trauma Informed Practice: A short guide for professionals working on the frontline*. London: Young Minds.

Gray, C., 1994. *Comic Strip Conversations*. Arlington: Future Horizons.

Gray, C., 2022. *Carol Gray Social Stories*. [Online] Available at: https://carolgraysocialstories.com/social-stories/ [Accessed 24 10 2022].

McCrory, E., n.d. *Childhood Trauma, the Brain and the Social World*. [Online] Available at: https://uktraumacouncil.org/resource/childhood-trauma-and-the-social-world [Accessed 13 07 2022].

National Autistic Society 2020 *Safeguarding young people on the autism spectrum*. [online] Available at https://www.autism.org.uk/shop/products/books-and-resources/safeguarding-young-people [Accessed 24 02 2023]

NSPCC, 2022. *Keeping Children Safe Online*. [Online] Available at: https://www.nspcc.org.uk/keeping-children-safe/online-safety/ [Accessed 26 10 2022].

Prizant, B. M., 2019. *A Different Way of Seeing Autism: Uniquely Human*. London: Souvenir Press.

Smith, A., Nanny, A., Hughes, J. & Wilshere, K., 2022. *The NEST Approach: Supporting Autistic Young People with Meltdowns*. [Online] Available at: https://www.barrierstoeducation.co.uk/meltdowns [Accessed 26 03 2023].

Spectrum Gaming, 2022a. *Autism and Trauma: A Neurodiversity Affirming Guide for Parents + Professionals*. [Online] Available at: https://www.barrierstoeducation.co.uk/trauma [Accessed 27 11 2022].

Taylor, J. L. & Corbett, B. A., 2014. A Review of Rhythm and Responsiveness of Cortisol in Individuals with Autism Spectrum Disorders. *Psychoneuroendocrinology*, 49, pp. 207–228.

Understanding Autism and Anxiety  (Spectrum Gaming, 2022b) https://www.barrierstoeducation.co.uk/anxiety

van Steensel, F. J. A., Perrin, S. & Bögels, S. M., 2011. Anxiety Disorders in Children and Adolescents with Autistic Spectrum Disorders: A Meta-Analysis. *Clinical Child and Family Psychology Review,* 17(3), pp. 302–17.

Ward, C. & Galpin, J., 2021. *The Anxiety Workbook for Supporting Teens Who Learn Differently: A Framework and Activities to Build Structural, Sensory and Social Certainty.* London: Jessica Kingsley Publishers.

# AUGMENTATIVE AND ALTERNATIVE COMMUNICATION

DOI: 10.4324/9781003154334-11

**Key points**

- Augmentative and alternative communication is anything that helps a child/young person with a communication difficulty to communicate more effectively.

**Focus on**

- Supporting people in the young person's settings to use aided language.
- Ensuring multi-modal communication is valued.
- Increasing communication opportunities.

## Introduction

Augmentative and alternative communication (AAC) is anything that helps a child/young person with a communication difficulty to communicate more effectively. This includes natural strategies that individuals have developed for themselves and strategies that have been taught to support their communication. These might include signing, symbol systems using core boards, communication books or voice output communication aids (VOCA). Any system introduced is used to **augment** the young person's communication, not to replace it. They will continue to use their effective strategies that are already working to extend their multi-modal communication.

A recent systematic review of the research evidence found positive effects of AAC used with autistic children and young adults on various measures, including communication and social outcomes (Hume et al., 2021).

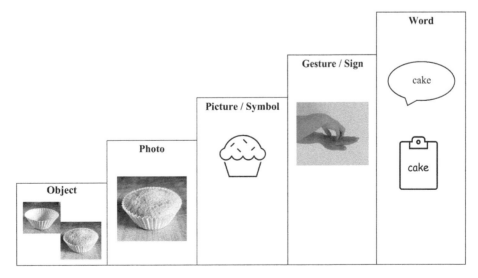

**FIGURE 9.1** Types of visual support.

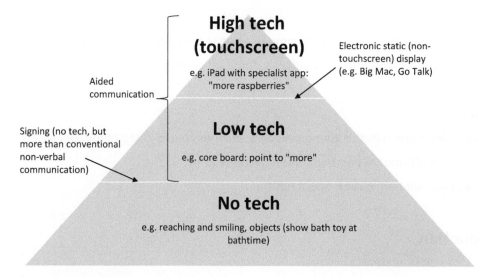

**FIGURE 9.2** Levels of AAC.

Autistic children who are not developing language effectively need to be supported and encouraged to use augmentative communication at an early stage. No-tech communication is often an early focus to support social communication and joint attention development.

A range of visual supports are used alongside spoken language (fig 9.1). Different children are helped by different types of support, as discussed in Chapter 5.

## No tech – what it is

No tech includes conventional non-verbal communication strategies such as using body language (including waving, pointing, reaching, pushing, grabbing, facial expression and proximity) and strategies that are encouraged or taught to support communication. These might include non-verbal and non-conventional communication, e.g. Makaton signing (makaton.org). See Chapter 5.

## Low tech – what it is

Using symbols, for example, the Picture Exchange Communication System® (PECS) (Pyramid Educational Consultants®, n.d.), a core board, language board or communication book e.g. Pragmatic Organisation Dynamic Display [PODD©] is a type of communication book (CPEC, n.d.).

## High tech – what it is

High-tech AAC includes iPads/tablets with specialist apps (e.g. Proloquo2Go, PODD), providing voice output (speech generating devices). This gives the child/young person a voice, and the app can support the young person's developing symbolic understanding as the link between symbol and spoken word is consolidated consistently.

**Starting AAC:** there are no precursors to the introduction of AAC. No skills are needed as a prerequisite to the introduction of AAC. A child/young person who is not following a typical communication developmental pathway must be introduced to support for their communication at an early stage. This is to *augment* their communication skills, whatever they may be.

However, awareness of a young person's symbolic understanding impacts decision-making. Using fixed symbol positions such as on a core board, language board or communication book can help a young person to learn the meaning of symbols, particularly for more abstract (core) vocabulary where the symbol is not easily recognisable.

Low tech is a vital backup to any high-tech system (batteries run out, screens break, devices crash). A low-tech system is essential so that the youngster always has a way to express themselves.

Low tech is often used to introduce communication aids and teach children and young people an understanding of symbols.

Symbols can and should be used to support language for a range of purposes. A core board helps provide a vocabulary set that will enable young people and their communication partners to express a range of functions.

Many families of children and young people with autism are keen to explore high-tech possibilities to support their non-speaking child/young person, particularly where the youngster is especially skilled at navigating their way around computers and tablets/iPads. In the last ten years, these have become increasingly accessible, so mainstream devices such as iPads can have highly specialist apps to support communication. This availability means that while this tech is widely available, decision-making may be based on availability rather than needs, and expertise to support the implementation of AAC is not necessarily in place. It can be a complex part of the role of the speech and language therapist (SLT) to support the young person's family in understanding the strengths and limitations of AAC.

Families understandably feel that if their child could talk, many of their difficulties would be resolved, and an iPad appears to be the solution. It is helpful to consider the young person's competencies and associated needs:

## Light's model

Light's model (1989) remains helpful in identifying competencies.

## Linguistic competence

(How) Is the child/young person communicating symbolically?

Children and young people who have not developed language following a typical pathway may have had far less exposure to the language that they are using. In particular, where they are learning to use visual systems, they are extremely unlikely to have been immersed in the linguistic environment they are learning (i.e. a symbol system), which will impact their progress. They are also limited to the symbols that someone else has selected for them, rather than having access to all the words that they have been exposed to through speech.

## Operational competence

How is a youngster able to access and operate a device? Do they have/respond to a contact point? Joint attention? Visual attention (scanning)? Sustained attention to navigation while searching/page turning?

Often, autistic children and young people have good technical skills with high-tech devices: able to operate mobile phones, laptops and tablets, remember passwords and navigate the internet to find preferred games or music independently, despite sometimes having limited language and learning ability. Their parents, teacher, relatives and siblings often identify these strengths and are keen to exploit their expert capabilities, using these strengths to support their weaker communication skills.

## Social competence

Does the youngster have a desire to communicate and communicative confidence?

The barrier for many autistic children learning to use any communication system appears to be initiation and motivation. Cause-effect play, people games and finally box exchanges are good first steps to teaching a child to give an item to another person to make something happen.

AAC may also benefit some autistic children and young people who find communication socially challenging but do not have specific language difficulties. They may be able to access communication using AAC when they cannot respond verbally due to high anxiety. For example, non-specialist apps on a phone can be used to take the pressure off verbal communication e.g. free text to speech apps.

## Strategic competence

Does the youngster have compensatory strategies and persistence?

The individual must use a combination of skills to communicate a message. Without good integration of the skills, communication may be ineffective despite some sophisticated skills.

Aaron had no spoken language but used symbols and body language to express himself relatively limitedly, mainly to meet his needs and immediate wishes. However, when an iPad with Proloquo2Go was introduced, he could use his excellent IT skills to quickly navigate the programme. He was socially motivated enough to comment **spontaneously**, e.g. finding his way to "flowers" (requiring navigating through several screens) at the garden centre. He remains relatively limited in his spontaneous use of language for a range of reasons, although this has increased to include commenting, clarifying, negotiating and joking. The iPad has also meant that interactions have been sustained for longer periods with a familiar conversational partner.

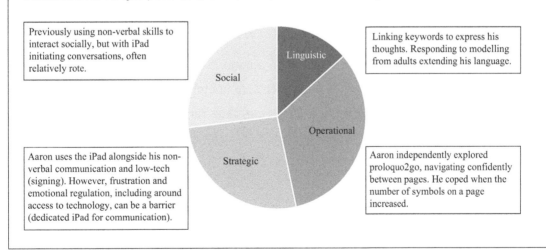

Previously using non-verbal skills to interact socially, but with iPad initiating conversations, often relatively rote.

Linking keywords to express his thoughts. Responding to modelling from adults extending his language.

Aaron uses the iPad alongside his non-verbal communication and low-tech (signing). However, frustration and emotional regulation, including around access to technology, can be a barrier (dedicated iPad for communication).

Aaron independently explored proloquo2go, navigating confidently between pages. He coped when the number of symbols on a page increased.

Core vocabulary: AAC

In this chapter, "core vocabulary" refers to the core words used on an AAC system, not the approach used to support children with an inconsistent speech disorder, which is also described as the core vocabulary approach.

## Core vocabulary

A core vocabulary allows a large variety of language to be expressed with a relatively small core vocabulary selected from studies of typical language use. However, it is also essential to include developmentally and personally relevant vocabulary as these may not have sufficient prominence in core vocabulary lists for early symbolic communicators (Laubscher & Light, 2020).

Most children who learn verbal language benefit from the modelling of spoken language from birth. Children and young people learning to use a symbol-based system rely on learning to use a system that has not been modelled from birth and is not in incidental use around them. Limited joint attention may also impact the young person's ability to benefit from incidental learning opportunities unless the focus of the modelling is specifically on the young person's focus of attention.

## What to do

Introduce a core board with as many symbols as the young person can cope with. Consider their visual attention and symbolic understanding. The more symbols on a page, the fewer pages will be needed in a book/device. Colour coding helps users navigate the board and helps support linking words and understanding the structure of language.

---

Symbols on a page...

Consideration of the number of symbols on a page is essential. It is often appropriate to be optimistic about the young person's competence, but a careful balance is needed: the more symbols on a page, the fewer page turns required, so the concentration demands are reduced. However, too many symbols can be overwhelming for the young person and their communication partners, resulting in slow progress and discouragement.

Consider hiding/fading out symbols that will be added later to a bigger grid.

---

## Modelling across the day: aided language

As the communication partner talks, point to the keywords. Symbols need to be modelled across the day. It is unrealistic to expect an autistic young person with significant communication needs to be able to learn to express themselves using a system that they have not seen in use and have not been taught to use.

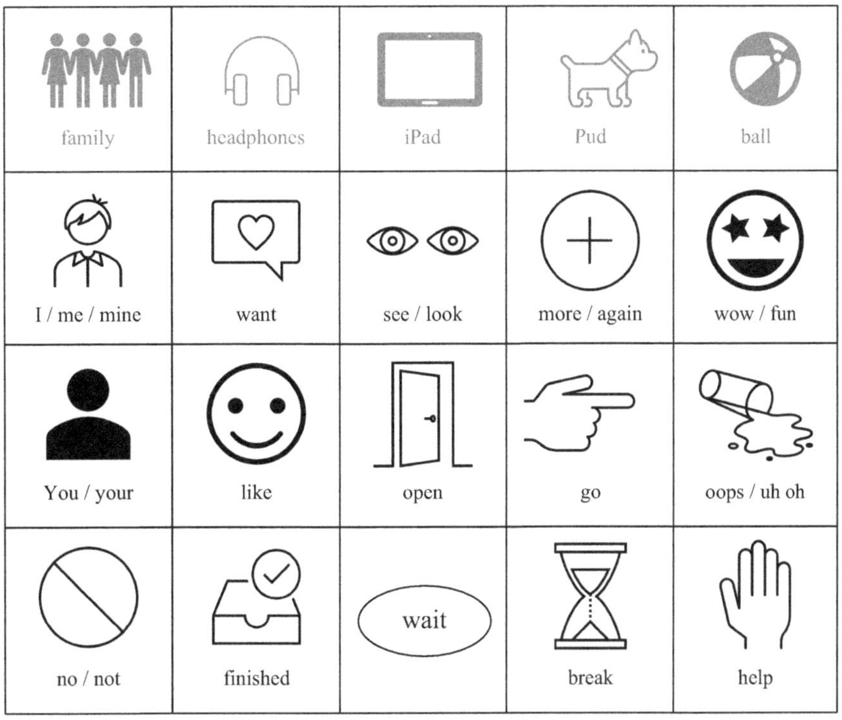

| | | | | |
|---|---|---|---|---|
| family | headphones | iPad | Pud | ball |
| I / me / mine | want | see / look | more / again | wow / fun |
| You / your | like | open | go | oops / uh oh |
| no / not | finished | wait | break | help |

**FIGURE 9.3** Core board with developmentally/personally relevant vocabulary (grey symbols).

Consider having a focus word and using the same word in different contexts: "<u>open</u> the door," "the blinds are <u>open</u>," "help <u>open</u> the crisps," "it's cold, the window's <u>open</u>," "<u>open</u> the paint," "oops, I left it <u>open</u>," "is the shop <u>open</u>?" "<u>open</u> your eyes!" "the box is not <u>open</u>," "the egg cracks <u>open</u> and a caterpillar comes out," "the chrysalis <u>opens</u> and a butterfly comes out," "the butterfly <u>opens</u> its wings."

PrAACtical AAC offer "A Year of Core Vocabulary Words" (Zangari, 2013) to develop the theme.

A research review of AAC modelling intervention (aided language) demonstrated that gains included: pragmatics, increases in communication turns and semantics, increases in expressive and receptive vocabulary, as well as increases in linking symbols and targeted morphology usage (Sennott et al., 2016).

---

**AIDED LANGUAGE SUPPORT**

Adults model using symbols to communicate a wide range of communication reasons in different situations. The purpose is to expose the young person to the symbols; imitation is not the goal.

---

Use familiar and preferred activities to reinforce particular and useful core vocabulary. For example:

- Play with cars: <u>look</u> fast!  – <u>Wow!</u> – <u>Uh oh</u>....
- Bubbles: wait – open – go – look – oops – like – fun.
- Playground: wait – look – go – fun – stop – finished.
- Breakfast: what do you <u>want</u>? – <u>look</u> we've got shreddies – <u>oops</u> I spilled the milk – do you <u>want</u> more – you <u>like</u> shreddies! – breakfast is <u>finished</u> – let's <u>go</u>.

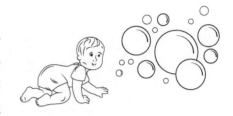

- Story: this could be a story you read or a video story (where the story is online).
- Games: board games, actions game (Pop Up Pirate, Mr Potato Head), playground games, etc.

A review of research found that successful strategies for developing a range of communicative functions in autistic children using AAC included teaching skills in structured, context-bound routines and prompting (Logan et al., 2022).

Specialist vocabulary can be added to the core page or as additional pages in a communication book. Ensure the core vocabulary is always available.

A voice output communication aid gives a young person a voice. The voice output also helps reinforce meanings as the youngster hears the word when they touch the symbol.

Autistic children and young people who use symbols to communicate and are introduced to a high-tech device are usually able to learn to use the device to request something they want. As with everyone, motivation is the most critical factor. Many young people need significant support to use other communicative functions.

> Kai was introduced to an iPad with Proloquo2Go with a 7 by 11 core vocabulary. While he did not use most of the core page despite modelling a range of vocabulary, he spontaneously requested "I want ice lolly" on a hot day!

Any/all communication forms (e.g. body language, facial expression, vocalisation, aided systems) can be used as part of a youngster's communication system and should be nurtured. The tendency is to use the easiest method so that a young person might have a clear and well-established "no" sign, and this will be used and should be accepted. They should not be required to use their aided AAC to express this when they already have an easy and efficient way to express "no."

AAC can powerfully support communication using aided language input, providing the child/young person with the benefit of symbols support alongside spoken language to enhance communication *without expecting the child/young person to point to symbols themselves.* This may rely greatly on the skills and interpretation of the communication partner, carefully watching the youngster's total communication (Sheldon, 2019).

## Summary

- There are no precursors to the introduction of AAC.
- AAC is used as part of the child/young person's "toolkit" to augment their communication.
- Aided language support is important to help youngsters learn how to use AAC, and it can be an effective communication support in itself as part of a total communication approach.

## Useful resources

www.communicationmatters.org.uk: Communication Matters is a charity that supports people of all ages who find it difficult to communicate as they have little or no clear speech.

www.praacticalaac.org: lots of practical ideas to support the implementation of AAC.

www.assistiveware.com includes Proloquo2Go information, plus blogs to support the implementation of AAC.

*What is PODD?* (Sheldon and Barthère, 2019) A powerful description of the impact of using aided language on communication.

## References

CPEC, n.d. *PODD: What Is PODD.* [Online] Available at: https://www.cpec.org.au/podd [Accessed 24 02 2023].

Hume, K. et al., 2021. Evidence-Based Practices for Children, Youth, and Young Adults with Autism: Third Generation Review. *Journal of Autism and Developmental Disorders*, 51, pp. 4013-4032.

Laubscher, E. & Light, J., 2020. Core Vocabulary Lists for Young Children and Considerations for Early Language Development: A Narrative Review. *Augmentative and Alternative Communication*, 36(1), pp. 43-53.

Light, J., 1989. Toward a Definition of Communicative Competence for Individuals using Augmentative and Alternative Communication Systems. *Augmentative and Alternative Communication*, 5(2), pp. 137-144.

Logan, K. A., Iacono, T. A. & Trembath, D., 2022. A Systematic Search and Appraisal of Intervention Characteristics Used to Develop Varied Communication Functions in Children with Autism Who Use Aided AAC. *Research in Autism Spectrum Disorders*, 90, pp. 51-64.

Pyramid Educational Consultants®, n.d. *What Is PECS®*. [Online] Available at: https://pecs-unitedkingdom.com/pecs/ [Accessed 29 09 2022].

Sennott, S. C., Light, J. C. & McNaughton, D., 2016. AAC Modeling Intervention Research Review. *Research and Practice for Persons with Severe Disabilities*, 41, pp. 101-115.

Sheldon, E., 2019. *What Is PODD*. [Online] Available at: https://www.assistiveware.com/blog/what-is-podd [Accessed 15 09 2022].

Zangari, C. C., 2013. *A Year of Core Vocabulary Words*. [Online] Available at: https://praactical.org/praactical/a-year-of-voucabulary-words/.

# Index

Note: Page numbers in *italics* indicate figures, and page numbers in **bold** indicate tables

T - #0004 - 090625 - C0 - 297/210/12 - SB - 9780367723149 - Matt Lamination